Chanc

DO NOT REMOVE.

ESSENTIAL DIAGNOSTIC TESTS

A guide to important principles
for nurses and laboratory technicians

Essential
Diagnostic Tests
in Biochemistry and
Haematology

P. T. Lascelles M.D. M.R.C.Path.
D. Donaldson M.R.C.P. M.R.C.Path.

MTP
MEDICAL AND TECHNICAL PUBLISHING CO LTD
1970

Published by

MTP

MEDICAL AND TECHNICAL PUBLISHING CO LTD
Chiltern House, Oxford Road, Aylesbury, Bucks

Copyright © 1971, P. T. Lascelles and
D. Donaldson

SBN 852 0001 46

First published 1971

Books in the "Essential knowledge" series for
nurses:

Essential Anatomy

Essential Medicine

Essential Physics, Chemistry and Biology

**Essential Biochemistry, Endocrinology and
Nutrition**

Essential Diagnostic Tests

Essential Physiology

PRINTED IN GREAT BRITAIN BY
THE GARDEN CITY PRESS LIMITED
LETCHWORTH, HERTFORDSHIRE

THIS SERIES REPRESENTS A NEW APPROACH TO the education of nurses, and medical laboratory technicians. Each volume has been written by a leading expert who is in close touch with the education of nurses.

These books do not cover any particular examination syllabus but each one contains more than enough information to enable the student to pass his or her examinations in that subject. The aim is rather to provide the understanding which will enable each person to get the most out of and put the most into his or her profession. Throughout we have tried to present medical science in a clear, concise and logical way. All the authors have endeavoured to ensure that students will truly understand the various concepts instead of having to memorize a mass of ill-digested facts. The message of this new series is that medicine is now moving away from the poorly understood dogmatism of not so very long ago. Many aspects of bodily function in health and disease can now be clearly and logically appreciated: what is required of the good nurse or paramedical worker is a thoughtful understanding and not a parrot-like memory.

Each volume is designed to be read in its own right. However, four titles: *Physics, Chemistry and Biology*; *Anatomy*; *Biochemistry, Endocrinology and Nutrition* and *Physiology* provide the foundations on which all the other books are based. The student who has read these four will get much more out of the other books which relate to clinical matters.

We hope that a feature of this series will be regular revision. Critical comments from readers will be much appreciated as these will help us to improve later editions.

Contents

ACKNOWLEDGEMENT

The authors wish to thank Dr. N. R. M. BUIST and the Editor of the British Medical Journal for permission to reproduce part of an article in appendix H on 'Screening Tests for Inborn Errors of Metabolism'.

1

Introduction

The aim of this guide is to provide both nurses and laboratory technicians with an up-to-date account of current diagnostic biochemical tests. A number of investigations which lie on the border-line of biochemistry and haematology are also included. There are many excellent books both in Great Britain and the United States which deal with the broader aspects of diagnostic tests (Ref. 1) but such is the complexity of modern medicine that it is necessary to provide a more specialized book incorporating the latest advances in practical biochemical and haematological investigations which are of diagnostic importance.

The present work has been designed as a reference book giving not only a large amount of factual data in a readily accessible form but also guidance on the interpretation of tests. It is hoped that it will be helpful to students not only in day to day problems in general and metabolic wards and laboratories but also in preparing for examinations. A considerable number of sections, giving greater detail and including rarer conditions, have been included for those who wish to read more deeply and a number of selected references have been added at the end of the book to open the way to further reading. Many common and important conditions which are not diagnosable by biochemical tests are not of course included.

Chapter 2 deals with general principles and it is hoped that this will be of particular value to ward staff. It is devoted mainly to details of how patients should be prepared or specimens collected for biochemical investigations.

Chapter 3 is intended as a fairly comprehensive reference section for the interpretation of individual tests. There has been some grouping of investigations which often go together under general headings such as 'electrolytes' and 'enzymes', but references to the specific tests under such headings can be readily obtained as they are arranged in alpha-betical order. Normal ranges are quoted together with the causes of raised and lowered values. Details of how function tests are carried out and the contra-indications to them are also given.

In Chapter 4 tests are grouped according to the patient's clinical diagnosis. Thus if a patient is suspected of suffering from, say, diabetic coma, all the biochemical investigations of diagnostic importance are listed under this heading. This section will be particularly useful in indicating further tests that are likely to be requested. It is hoped that this and the preceding section will be of value not only to nursing staff but also to laboratory technicians in helping them to appreciate the clinical significance of the tests with which they are concerned.

The appendices are intended for quick reference and contain specific details on the preparation of patients and on the collection of specimens including those from patients suspected of having been poisoned.

An appendix is also included on 'ward side-room testing'. In some hospitals there is a tendency nowadays for less side-room tests to be carried out on the ward than previously. Nevertheless, they provide an important part of the training of student nurses. Outside hospitals they are becoming increasingly important in group general practice.

Finally, some explanation is necessary concerning the sections on intravenous fluid therapy and tube feeding. These do not come within the scope of diagnostic procedures but on account of their close association with the 'biochemical status' of patients, their inclusion has been thought justified.

2

General principles

A biochemical test consists of the measurement under specified conditions of some parameter (usually the concentration of a substance in a body fluid, e.g. creatinine in serum or its excretion in the urine during a 24 hour period) and a comparison of this is made with the normal. The result therefore (expressed in specific units, e.g. mg per 100 ml) may be interpreted as high, normal or low. The matter is not quite as simple as this however, as it is often not possible to say with certainty what the normal value is. Moreover, it is often possible for a patient who is clearly unwell to have a normal or near normal test while another patient with the same disease will have an abnormal result. (An analogy may be drawn with the body temperature. Some patients with, say, bronchopneumonia will have a high temperature while others during some stage of the same disease may have a normal temperature.) A further complication is that occasionally healthy subjects will show an abnormal response to a test.

As a general principle it is important to perform a battery of tests, e.g. liver function tests, and to repeat them at intervals. By observing the changing pattern of responses, valuable information may be obtained concerning the progress of a disease process.

The normal range

If one takes a group of healthy subjects and measures some parameter, e.g. blood urea, one will obtain a scatter of results, but it will soon become clear that most of the results lie between say 20 mg/100 ml and 40 mg/100 ml and one may therefore say that the normal range is 20–40 mg/100 ml.

The mean and standard deviation are figures which may be derived mathematically from a group of results and which have certain properties which are useful when making comparisons between different groups of results.

The scatter of results however, is often not even throughout this range, and the figures instead of showing a 'normal distribution' (Fig. 1), may show a 'lognormal distribution' (Fig. 2).

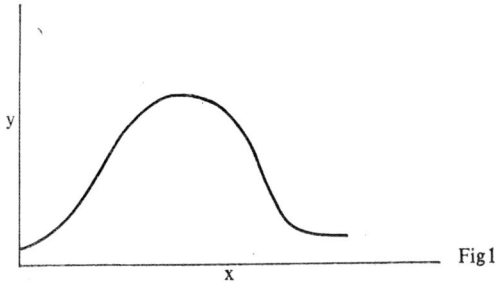

Fig 1

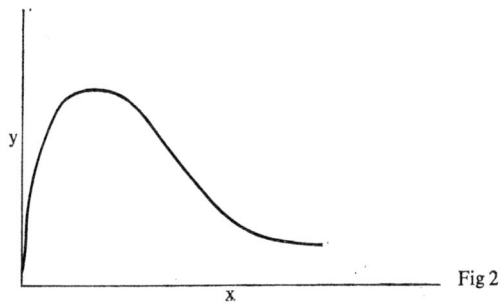

Fig 2

The practical importance of this lies in the fact that a result slightly outside one limit of the normal range will be of much greater significance than another result equally removed from the other limit.

In addition to the patient's disease, many factors, both physical and emotional, will affect the results of tests. For example it is known that simply bringing a patient into hospital will affect the plasma cortisol level. Thus the normal range for healthy subjects will often be of no value for the assessment of hospital in-patients.

Other factors affecting the normal range include age, sex, race and diet, moreover a different range of normal values is required for many tests carried out during pregnancy. The results of many investigations are influenced in addition by the time of day, whether or not the patient is fasting, whether at rest or after exercise and in a few instances whether recumbent or standing.

The normal range is also critically dependant upon the analytical technique employed by the laboratory and the form in which the specimen is collected, (e.g. venous or capillary blood) and in some cases the rapidity with which specimens are conveyed to the laboratory.

Collection of specimens

In some hospitals routine blood collections are made by the laboratory staff. The wards however always have the responsibility of preparing the patient and of supervising the collection of other specimens, particularly 24 hour urine samples, and of undertaking the despatch of specimens to the correct laboratory. Where blood samples are not collected by laboratory staff the ward will have to provide the correct blood containers.

The importance of the accurate collection and correct despatch of specimens cannot be over-emphasized. These procedures constitute a critical link between the patient and the final result of this test and if the initial collection is inaccurate or the sample is mishandled all subsequent analyses will be invalid.

Although in general these principles are well appreciated, yet so important are they that a number of practical points are worth emphasizing.

PREPARATION OF THE PATIENT. The patient should be advised that a test is to be carried out and at the very least a few brief details should be explained. It is general experience that patients are less frightened if they know roughly the nature of a test and how long it will last. In any case informing patients about tests helps to ensure their co-operation and gives them their fair right to refuse investigation in some instances.

For many biochemical tests it is necessary for the patient to fast from the night before, blood being collected early the following morning. Unless specifically indicated to the contrary these patients can usually be allowed to drink water (but not tea, milk or fruit juices) and in many instances water intake should be encouraged in order to ensure an adequate urine flow to facilitate the collection of urine specimens. Clearly these remarks do not apply if the laboratory instructions state 'Nil by mouth'.

In addition for some tests it is necessary for patients to have been on a special diet for several days before commencing the collection of specimens, and details of this diet will be included with the instructions for the test.

Generally most tests are performed with the patient resting in bed. He may be allowed up to toilet first thing in the morning and then return to lie quietly in bed. For some tests however (e.g. Basal Metabolic Rate (B.M.R.) and blood lactate assays) *complete bed rest* is essential and preferably in a quiet single room (essential for B.M.R.). In a very few instances (e.g. prolonged fast with blood glucose determinations for the assessment of hypoglycaemia) it is important for the patient not to be at rest during the test.

TAKING BLOOD SAMPLES. Blood is withdrawn from a vein, usually from the ante-cubital fossa in the front of the arm. A tourniquet is applied to the upper arm with sufficient pressure to impede the return of blood from the hand while at the same time not being sufficiently tight to prevent arterial blood from entering the arm. (Approximately 90–110 mm of mercury if a sphygmomanometer is used—this is often useful in patient with poor veins.) The tourniquet should be applied for the minimum of time (e.g. 30 seconds) prior to blood taking and released immediately afterwards. In some instances (e.g. serum calcium assay and blood lactate assay) use of a tourniquet may invalidate the results. Remove the needle before gently transferring blood to the container.

If capillary blood is being collected from a finger prick or lobe of ear the application of excessive local pressure in an attempt to increase the flow of blood will seriously affect the results.

Femoral vein, jugular vein and arterial punctures are occasionally carried out by medical personnel and require special knowledge and techniques.

URINE COLLECTION. *Early morning specimens.* For biochemical tests it is frequently necessary to obtain part of the first specimen of urine passed in the morning, and this is usually collected into a clean universal container. Unless specifically stated it is not necessary to collect the whole specimen, but if urine volume measurements are being charted on a patient even the small volume of early morning specimens (approximately 20 ml in a universal container) must be accounted for on the charts. Unless the specimen is being sent for bacteriological examination it is not necessary to collect a midstream specimen nor to use a sterile container.

Consecutive random specimens. If consecutive random specimens are being collected from a patient with or without an indwelling catheter it is imperative to ensure that the bladder is completely emptied between collections. Thus the residual urine left in an incompletely emptied bladder in a patient with diabetic coma may still contain glucose even when the patient has been rendered hypoglycaemic and this could result in the wrong treatment being administered.

24 hour urine collection. It is often convenient for ward staff to commence 24 hour urine collections at, say, 8 a.m., particularly if this coincides with the commencement of fluid balance charts. However, 24 hour urine collections may in fact commence at any time, the really important point being that the timing and collection should be *accurate.*

At the given time, say 10 a.m., the patient passes urine and the specimen is discarded. It is essential that the patient be told to empty the bladder completely, and where possible not while lying in bed, and if collections are being made from patients with an indwelling catheter gentle suprapubic pressure should be applied. All urine passed sub sequently should be placed carefully into the bottle provided. Thus the first specimen to be placed into the bottle marked 10 a.m. in the example quoted may well be at 1 p.m. This is correct because although the bladder voids urine intermittently the kidneys, of course, secrete it continuously and the specimen voided at 1 p.m. began to accumulate in the bladder at 10 a.m.

The patient is instructed to end the test by passing the last specimen into the bottle at 10 a.m. the following morning. It is essential that all timing should be precise, although this may present problems in a busy ward. It is no use starting or ending a collection *even a few minutes early or late.* In order to help the patient empty the bladder at precisely the correct time it is often helpful to suggest that urine is not voided for, say, one to two hours before the end of the test. Thus. again in the example quoted, the patient should not pass urine on the second day at 9 a.m. because he might then find difficulty in passing it again at 10 a.m.

Occasionally, however, particularly with neurological patients. there may be a genuine difficulty in passing urine at the correct time. Under these circumstances the patient should pass the urine as near as possible to the correct time *but the exact time must be noted* and the bottle labelled appropriately, e.g. 23 hour and 35 minute specimen, 24 hour and 20 minute specimen instead of 24 hour precise specimen. This is not as satisfactory as the correct 24 hour sample but some allowance may then be made by the laboratory which is not otherwise possible.

It is important to remember that frequently the urine collection bottle will contain chemicals for preservation of the urine, and these must not be emptied out. They may take the form of organic solvents (e.g. toluene) or inorganic acids (e.g. dilute sulphuric acid), and patients, particularly out-patients, should be warned that these chemicals may impart an odour to the bottle or be dangerous if allowed to come into contact with the skin. It may be noted that even an appreciable volume of aqueous preservative (e.g. 20 ml) will give rise to no error at all in the 24 hour collection, for although it will dilute the urine it will also increase the urine volume by a similar amount; thus calculations based on the whole 24 hour urine volume will be accurate.

Finally, particularly in the case of out-patients, it is imperative to provide sufficient bottles for the whole collection. Nothing is more irritating to laboratory staff than to receive a so-called complete 24 hour urine sample that just happens to fill the bottle exactly!

If several 24 hour samples are being collected consecutively the patient may go straight on to the second 24 hours after completing the first.

Short period urine collections particularly for clearance tests. It is sometimes necessary to collect all urine passed over relatively short periods of time, e.g. 30 minutes or 2 hours, particularly in association with clearance tests. Exactly the same principles apply as for the 24 hour urine collection but even greater accuracy is needed here. The bladder must be emptied completely and all timings made to *an accuracy of at least 1 minute.* Experience shows that one member of staff must be delegated to supervise such collections in order to avoid inaccuracies and the inevitable waste of time necessitated by having to repeat these tests.

COLLECTION OF STOOLS FOR FAECAL ANALYSIS. An absolute minimum of 4 days collection, and preferably 5, 6 or 7 days collection should be made in the case of faecal fat. All specimens should be collected into cellophane and placed in containers. Again, as in urine collection, if the patient is unable to produce a specimen at the required time, *the accurate timing* of the final specimen when it is passed will always be possible. The use of an oral marker such as carmine increases accuracy, though increasing use is being made of the administration orally of an accurately known amount of chromium sesquioxide. In this event the final result is expressed not in terms of the total stool passed but as a ratio, e.g. fat/chromium sesquioxide, and has the advantage that if one specimen is lost an accurate result can still be obtained.

Laxatives should be avoided during stool collection for biochemical tests.

COLLECTION OF OTHER BIOCHEMICAL MATERIAL INCLUDING CEREBROSPINAL FLUID (CSF). These, which include aspirated fluids (e.g. pleural fluid), are collected by the medical staff and should be placed in clean dry bottles containing no preservative. In most instances bacteriological examinations will also be required in addition to biochemical tests and sterile procedures and bottles will be required. In the case of CSF collection into two bottles is necessary. This is not only prevents complete loss of the specimen in the event of one bottle being broken, but it also enables the laboratory to say whether any blood present is mainly in the first bottle or evenly mixed. In the first instance, the cause would be local bleeding produced by the lumbar puncture; the second would point to subarachnoid haemorrhage.

Two further points merit special consideration. Firstly, biopsy specimens (including those obtained in the operating theatre) which are being taken for biochemical analysis (as opposed to histological analysis) should **never** be placed in Formalin or saline, but rather into clean dry containers.

The second point also concerns biopsy specimens particularly those obtained at operations. General speaking, relatively complicated analyses are required and prior arrangements with the laboratory must be made. Often the specimen may have to be taken **at once** into a thermos flask containing carbon dioxide snow and sent immediately to the person concerned for analysis.

DISPOSAL OF SPECIMENS. Once a specimen has been accurately collected, attention must be given to its proper disposal and despatch to the laboratory.

It is sound general principle to assume that most specimens will not be stable even for a short period if left standing in the ward. For example, it is quite often necessary to centrifuge blood immediately in order to separate the cells from plasma. Every bottle or tube must be sealed with the proper stopper or lid and if it contains preservative or anti-coagulant gently inverted two or three times to mix. This does not apply to clean dry containers with a cork stopper and in a few special cases to be listed later, and also if blood samples are being collected under liquid paraffin for alkali reserve estimation. *No specimens should ever be shaken.*

It is of course mandatory that specimens be accurately labelled. Full details should be given including the hospital number. Specimens for forensic laboratories will require special handling and labelling.

Specimens requiring special attention (e.g. blood for pyruvate or lactate assay) will normally be collected by the laboratory staff, pipetted at the bedside and placed at once into Thermos flasks containing ice. Other specimens should be sent to the laboratory as soon as possible and centrifuged within 1 hour of collection. If they do remain in the wards for short periods they should never be allowed to stand near radiators or in bright sunlight. Specimens of all types obtained during hours when the laboratory is 'closed' should be placed at once in a specially designated refrigerator at 4°C or in a cold room also at 4°C. Rarely specimens may need to go straight into the 'deep freeze' refrigerator at $-20°C$ in the laboratory.

During 'normal working hours' however, specimens should be sent directly to the laboratory office as early as possible during the day and left in charge of a responsible person. It is important that specimens should arrive early for although automated analyses have solved some laboratory problems, the arrival of the occasional late specimen still entails a great deal of extra work in the laboratory.

Radioactive samples

Radioactive isotopes are not infrequently given to patients either for therapeutic purposes (e.g. phosphorus 32 for the treatment of Polycythaemia Vera) or for diagnostic purposes (e.g. Technecium 99M for brain scanning or Iodine[131] and Iodine [132] for assessment of thyroid function). In the case of isotopes used in radiotherapy large doses are administered and special precautions in the ward will be necessary but these do not lie within the scope of this book. In the case of radio-isotopes used for diagnostic tests no special precautions are necessary during the collection of specimens as the doses are small. If however a specimen of, say, radioactive urine is spilled, the radiological protection officer should be notified.

Tolerance tests

Although it is necessary to collect many samples for diagnostic biochemical tests with the patient under basal conditions, i.e. fasting and at rest, further important information can be obtained by observing a patient's biochemical response to standardized 'stress' situations, either physical (for example after exercise) or biochemical (for example after an oral glucose load or an intravenous insulin injection). Such investigations form the basis of tolerance tests. Most physiological functions are carried out with a considerable degree of reserve, and tolerance tests are designed to measure the amount of reserve function present. The importance of this lies in the fact that many disease processes will, in the early stages, reduce the amount of reserve function before producing symptoms that the patient may notice. Thus early diagnosis lies in detecting and measuring this decrease in reserve function. A good example is seen in the detection of diabetes mellitus. In the late stages of diabetes, particularly in diabetic coma the patient will have a high blood sugar at all times. However, a glucose tolerance test will reveal an abnormal response in the early stages of diabetes when the fasting blood glucose may still be within normal limits. A further extension of this principle is found in the cortisone-stressed glucose tolerance test. Here a normal glucose tolerance test may be repeated after the administration of cortisone. In very early diabetes mellitus the glucose tolerance test itself may be normal or very nearly so but when repeated after 'stressing' the patient with cortisone will become clearly abnormal. Many other examples of this important principle will be described later.

Clearance tests

The term clearance refers to the theoretical volume of blood which is totally cleared of a given compound in unit time. It entails the simultaneous measurement of blood and urine concentrations of the compound under investigation together with the measurement of urine volume over a specified period of time. It is an important index of excretory function, but it should be appreciated that it is only a theoretical index as many compounds are not in fact totally cleared from the blood.

Request forms

These are filled in by the medical staff and must contain adequate clinical details as well as all data necessary for patient recognition, particularly the hospital number. Generally speaking it is helpful for the laboratory if one request form accompanies each investigation even if this is to be repeated on successive days. Separate request forms and often a letter are of course necessary for investigations which are being carried out in separate laboratories.

Units of measurement

These are defined in the glossary.

Generally speaking blood constituents are expressed in mg/100 ml or mEq/litre, the latter being a more meaningful term in the relation of one constituent to another.

Haemoglobin values are now usually expressed in grams/100 ml rather than percentage.

Most urine constituents are expressed as the amount excreted per 24 hours. In many instances this figure is influenced by the patient's diet; consequently the limits of normal are frequently wide.

Osmolality is expressed in mOsmols/kg (of water), this figure being slightly more accurate than mOsmols/litre.

Enzyme activity should now always be expressed as International Units per litre.

Results of clearance tests are expressed as ml/minute. As mentioned above this is the theoretical volume of blood completely cleared of the constituent under consideration.

Blood for grouping and crossmatching

Of all laboratory tests, the one in which it is of vital importance to pay attention to detail, is when blood is being collected for grouping and crossmatching. The result of the laboratory tests determine the group of the blood which is eventually given directly to the patient should he subsequently require a transfusion. If the wrong group is given tragedy may result. It is therefore necessary to ensure that the blood for the test is collected from the right patient.

The patient must always be asked 'What is your name?' It is not satisfactory merely to say 'Are you Mr. Smith?' A deaf or confused patient is likely to say 'Yes' whatever is asked. In the case of an unconscious patient it is necessary to check with the Sister or Senior Staff Nurse in charge that he or she is the right patient. Again, it is not satisfactory to look at the temperature chart at the end of the bed for the name as the wrong chart may have been placed there.

10 ml of blood is withdrawn from the vein, and allowed to clot in the tube which must be correctly and fully labelled *immediately*, before it is placed elsewhere. The labelling must include the full name, case number, the date and the ward. An incorrectly labelled or unlabelled specimen will not be accepted by the laboratory.

An important consideration when requesting blood grouping and crossmatching, is that sufficient time is given to the laboratory staff for the test. *At least* 24 hours warning is required so that blood which may not be stocked at the laboratory can be obtained from the Regional Blood Transfusion centre. In the case of a rare group even longer time may be necessary. It is good practice to send blood for grouping on admission of the patient if it is known or suspected that he may subsequently have an operation which may necessitate blood transfusion, and to request grouping and retention of the serum in the laboratory. This means that when the date of operation is known it is not necessary to take further blood. The group of the patient can therefore be looked up in the file and the appropriate bottles selected for crossmatching, using the stored serum for the test. Note that Dextran therapy may interfere with grouping and cross matching.

It takes about 2 hours to group a patient routinely (A B O and rhesus groups), and a similar time for the crossmatch. It is possible, however, to shorten this procedure in an emergency, provided that the bottles selected are compatible with the patient.

The whole point of grouping and crossmatching is to ensure safety in blood transfusion, by detecting patients with rare antibodies and antigens, and if these are present to identify them and make available blood which is compatible. This may take several days and in certain rare cases much longer. It is therefore vital that as much warning as possible be given to the laboratory in order that it may function efficiently for the benefit of the patient, and that what should have been a routine procedure does not through lack of foresight become an emergency measure.

3

Index of diagnostic tests with normal values: important conditions in which they may be abnormal

This chapter is intended as a fairly comprehensive reference section for the interpretation of individual tests. Normal ranges are quoted together with the causes of raised and lowered values. Note that the abbreviations used are as follows:

N.R. = Normal Range   R = Raised   L = Lowered

BLOOD

BIOCHEMISTRY

Whole Blood (B), Plasma (P) and serum (S)

BICARBONATE (SPECIAL COLLECTION)
(*a.*) Alkali reserve (P).
N.R. 24–32 mEq/litre.
(*b.*) Standard bicarbonate (B).
N.R. 22·4–25·8 mEq/litre.
(*c*). Base excess (B).
N.R. (+2·3) mEq/litre—(−2·3) mEq/litre.
R. Metabolic alkalosis.
   Respiratory acidosis.

L. Metabolic acidosis.
   Respiratory alkalosis.

BROMIDE (Br^-) (S)
Therapeutic Range 10–30 mg/100 ml.
Intoxication > 100 mg/100 ml.

CALCIUM (Ca^{++}) (S)
N.R. 9·0–11·0 mg/100 ml. (4·5–5·5 mEq/litre.)
R. Primary hyperparathyroidism. There is no fall in the serum
   calcium after cortisone therapy.
   Sarcoidosis.
R. Myelomatosis, carcinomatosis of bone, vitamin D intoxication.
   Excessive intake of alkalis with milk (milk-alkali syndrome).
L. Hypoparathyroidism. Pseudohypoparathyroidism.
   Rickets and osteomalacia.
   Malabsorption syndrome.
(In all these conditions tetany may be present.)

COPPER (Cu^{+++}) (SPECIAL COLLECTION)
N.R. 90–120 µg/100 ml.
R. Many forms of anaemia. Leukaemia and lymphomas.
L. Wilson's disease.
   Nephrotic syndrome.
   Kwashiorkor.

"CORTISOL" (11-HYDROXYCORTICOSTEROIDS)
(SPECIAL COLLECTION)
N.R. Depends on the time of day (diurnal variation), levels being highest at 8 a.m.
falling to lowest at 12 midnight.
8 a.m. 5–15 µg/100 ml.
R. Cushings' syndrome (adrenocortical hyperplasia, adenoma,
   carcinoma of adrenal cortex, carcinoma of lung. Basophil
   adenoma of pituitary).
   Obesity.
   Cortisone drug therapy.
L. Addison's disease.
   Pituitary insufficiency (chromophobe adenoma).

CREATINE (S)
N.R. 0·2–0·6 mg/100 ml.
R. Muscle wasting disorders.
   Renal failure.
   Hyperthyroidism.
L. Not clinically important.

CREATININE (S)
N.R. 0·9–1·7 mg/100 ml.
R. Acromegaly and gigantism.
   Acute and chronic renal failure.
L. Not clinically significant.

ELECTROLYTES (P)
Chloride (Cl⁻)
N.R. 97–107 mEq/litre.
R. As for sodium but in addition respiratory alkalosis and metabolic acidosis.

L. As for sodium but in addition from prolonged vomiting or gastric aspiration.

Potassium (K⁺)
N.R. 3·6–5·4 mEq/litre.
R. Advanced renal failure.
   Too rapid replacement of potassium during therapy particularly intravenously in patients with renal failure or low urine output.
   Diabetic coma before treatment is commenced.
   Addison's disease.

L. Inadequate potassium replacement particularly in patients on I.V. therapy with high urine output.
   Diuretic therapy.
   Cushing's syndrome or administration of cortisone and similar drugs.
   Potassium losing nephritis.
   Gastro-intestinal fluid loss and diarrhoea.
   Periodic paralysis.

Sodium (Na⁺)
N.R. 133–148 mEq/litre.
R. Dehydration, e.g. water deprivation, diabetes insipidus.
   Over treatment with I.V. saline infusions.
   Cushing's syndrome or steroid administration.
   Rarely brain damage and disease (primary cerebral hyper-nitraemia).

L. Water intoxication (e.g. psychogenic water drinking, over treatment with I.V. 5 per cent glucose in water).
   Addison's disease and pituitary insufficiency.
   Inappropriate secretion of anti-diuretic hormone, e.g. some cases of lung carcinoma, porphyria.
   Gastro-intestinal fluid loss and diarrhoea.

ENZYMES (S)
Acid phosphatase (Formol-stable)
N.R. 0·5–5 I.U./litre.
R. Carcinoma of prostate gland.

L. Not clinically important.

Alkaline phosphatase
N.R. 20–90 I.U./litre.
R. Many forms of acute and chronic liver disease but particularly in the presence of biliary obstruction.
   Primary hyperparathyroidism.
   Paget's disease of bone.
   Healing fractures, vitamin D deficient rickets, and malabsorption syndrome.
   Renal failure with secondary hyperparathyroidism.
   Bone sarcoma.
   Myelomatosis.
   Carcinomatosis of bone.

L. Hypophosphatasia.

Amylase
N.R. 4,000 I.U./litre.
R. Acute pancreatitis.
   Mumps.
   Acute urinary suppression.

L. Not clinically important.

Caeruloplasmin (as measured by copper oxidase activity)
N.R. 23–44 mg/100 ml.
R. Pregnancy.
   After oral contraceptive drugs.

L. Wilson's disease.
   Kwashiorkor.
   Chronic liver disease.

Creatine phosphokinase (C.P.K.)
N.R. ♂ 10–66 I.U./litre.   ♀ 10–43 I.U./litre.
R. Duchenne muscular dystrophy, both severe progressive and benign slowly progressive (Becker) types.
   Affected carriers of both types.
   Autosomal recessive patients but not carriers of this type.
   Acute polymyositis and dermatomyositis.
   Limb girdle muscular dystrophy but not in carriers.
   Cardiac infarction.
   Crush injury of muscle.
   Hypothyroidism.

L. Not clinically important.

Glutamic-oxalacetic transaminase (G.O.T.) (alanine aminotransferase)
N.R. 2–20 I.U./litre.
R. This intracellular enzyme is raised in many conditions in which there is tissue destruction including:
Cardiac infarction
Acute pancreatitis
Liver necrosis due to infective hepatitis (acute or chronic)
Crush injury.
L. Not clinically important.

Glutamic-pyruvate transaminase (G.P.T.) (aspartate aminotransferase)
N.R. 2–15 I.U./litre.
R. Liver necrosis due to acute or chronic hepatitis.
L. Not clinically important.

α-hydroxybutyrate dehydrogenase (H.B.D.)
N.R. 56–125 I.U./litre.
R. Many forms of tissue damage but particularly in cardiac infarction.
L. Not clinically important.

Isocitrate dehydrogenase (I.C.D.)
N.R. 0·9–4·0 I.U./litre.
R. Infective hepatitis and glandular fever hepatitis.
Secondary carcinomatosis.
Drug hepatitis.
L. Not clinically important.

Lactate dehydrogenase
N.R. 145–375 I.U./litre.
R. Cardiac infarction.
Pulmonary infarction. (Iso-enzyme pattern different from cardiac infarction.)
Duchenne muscular dystrophy, haemolytic anaemias (and pernicious anaemia.)
L. Not clinically important.

5-Nucleotidase
N.R. 5–17 I.U./litre.
R. Many forms of acute and chronic liver disease but particularly in the presence of biliary obstruction.
L. Not clinically important.

FOLIC ACID (S)
N.R. 4–19 mμg/ml. (Value for red cells 80–470 mμg/ml.
R. Folic acid drug therapy.
  Pernicious anaemia.

L. Malabsorption syndromes.
  Dietary deficiency.
  Therapy with anticonvulsant and 'antifolic acid' drugs.
  Pregnancy.
  Chronic haemolytic anaemias, chronic leukaemias.

IODINE (PROTEIN BOUND) (P.B.I.) (S)
N.R. 4–8 μg/100 ml.
R. Thyrotoxicosis.
  Pregnancy.
  Oestrogen drug therapy (including oral contraceptives).
  Iodine containing compounds including medicines and radio-
    opaque contrast media.

L. Hypothyroidism primary or secondary to pituitary disease.
  Many forms of drug therapy including steroids.
  Nephrotic syndrome.
  Treatment with tri-iodothyronine.

IRON
Iron binding capacity (special collection)
N.R. 220–400 μg/100 ml.
R. Haemochomatosis.

L. Iron deficiency anaemia.

Serum iron (special collection)
N.R. 70–170 μg/100 ml.
R. Haemochomatosis.

L. Iron deficiency anaemia.

LACTATE (SPECIAL COLLECTION)
N.R. 6–18 mg/100 ml.
R. Familial lactic acidosis.

L. Failure to rise after ischemic exercise indicates muscle phosphory-
    lase deficiency (McArdle's syndrome) together with other
    muscle enzyme deficiencies (see Ischemic Exercise Lactate
    Test).
  Special precautions are necessary for the collection of blood
    samples.

LEAD (SPECIAL COLLECTION)
Whole blood should contain less than 50 μg/100 ml. High levels are associated with lead intoxication but intermediate levels may be encountered with exposure to lead without intoxication. The acceptable blood level in children is lower, i.e. 36 μg/100 ml.

Special precautions are necessary for the collection of blood samples.

LIPIDS (S)
Total cholesteral N.R. 140–250 mg/100 ml.
R. Diabetes mellitus.
  Biliary obstruction and primary biliary cirrhosis.
  Familial hypercholesterolaemia (several types).
  Nephrotic syndrome.
  Hypothyroidism.
  Pregnancy.
L. Hyperthyroidism.
  Severe liver damage.
  Primary lipoprotein deficiencies. a-β lipoproteinaemia, Tangier disease.

TRIGLYCERIDES
N.R. 25–150 mg/100 ml.
R. Familial hyperlipidaemia (except Fredrichson Type II).
  Tangier disease.
  Diabetes.
  Glycogen storage disease.
  Nephrosis.
  Pregnancy.
  Chronic liver disease.
L. a-β lipoproteinaemia.

MAGNESIUM (Mg^{++}) (S)
N.R. 1·5–1·8 mEq/litre.
R. Administration of magnesium salts (including magnesium sulphate enemas) to patients with impaired renal function.
L. Primary hyperaldosteronism which may be associated with tetany in the presence of a normal serum calcium.

OSMOLALITY (P)
N.R. 280–290 mOsmols/kg.
R. Diabetes insipidus.
  Any condition in which there is a raised plasma sodium sugar or urea.

L. Water intoxication, either due to psychogenic water drinking or over treatment with intravenous 5 per cent glucose in water. Any condition in which there is inappropriate secretion of anti-diuretic hormone; overdosage of vasopression.

OXYGEN (ARTERIAL BLOOD—SPECIAL COLLECTION)
PaO_2
N.R. 90–110 mm Hg.
R. Not clinically important.
L. Many diseases of the respiratory system including airways obstruction disease and disorders of gas transfer.
Congestive heart failure.

$PaCO_2$
N.R. 38–43 mm Hg.
R. Many diseases of respiratory system in which there is an inability to eliminate carbon dioxide. Underventilation.
L. Overventilation due to hysteria or during anaesthesia.

pH (ARTERIAL BLOOD—SPECIAL COLLECTION)
N.R. 7·37–7·42
R. Metabolic alkalosis.
Respiratory alkalosis.
L. Metabolic acidosis.
Respiratory acidosis.

PHOSPHORUS (P) (RESULTS EXPRESSED AS INORGANIC PHOSPHORUS)
N.R. *Adults:* 2·5–4·5 mg/100 ml.   *Children:* 4·0–6·0 mg/100 ml.
R. Advanced renal failure.
Hypoparathyroidism.
Active acromegaly.
L. Primary hyperarathyroidism.
Rickets and osteomalacia (both dietary and vitamin D resistant).
De Toni-Fanconi syndrome.
Chronic renal acidosis.
Phosphaturic rickets.

PROTEIN (S)
Total protein	N.R. 6·3–7·8 g/100 ml.
Albumin	N.R. 50%–65% of total protein
Globulin (Total)	N.R. 35%–50% of total protein
α_1 globulin	N.R. 1%–5% of total protein
α_2 globulin	N.R. 4·5%–9·5% of total protein
β globulin	N.R. 11·0%–16·0% of total protein
γ globulin	N.R. 14·0%–20·0% of total protein

The ratio of albumin to globulin varies in health between $1\cdot0/1\cdot0$–$1\cdot9/1\cdot0$. Each fraction may vary independently in disease but often there is an associated 'compensatory' change in the other fraction. Similarly the several globulin fractions may show variations giving rise to characteristic patterns in disease.

Albumin
R. Severe dehydration from any cause.
L. Neprotic syndrome.
   Severe acute and chronic liver disease.
   Burns.
   Ulcerative colitis.
   Severe malnutrition including kwashiorkor.

Total Globulin
R. Chronic liver disease.
   Secondary carcinomatosis of liver.
   Myelomatosis.
   Sarcoidosis.
   The collagen diseases.
L. Not clinically useful. More information can be obtained from a study of the individual globulin fractions.

α_1 *Globulin*
R. Nephritis.
   Collagen diseases.
   Any cause of tissue damage.

α_2 *Globulin*
R. Any cause of tissue damage, including malignant disease, collagen disease, sarcoidosis, liver disease and many forms of kidney, particularly in nephrotic syndrome.

β *Globulin*
R. Many forms of collagen disease and liver disease.
   Particularly high levels occur in myelomatosis, nephrotic syndrome and the hyperlipidaemias.

γ *Globulin*
R. Many forms of kidney and liver disease.
   Collagen disease, carcinomatosis, myelomatosis, sarcoidosis, kala-azar, macro and cryoglobulinaemia.

L. Congenital and acquired agammaglobulinaemia and secondary hypogammaglobulinaemia.

Fibrinogen (P)
N.R. 200–400 mg/100 ml.
R. Acute infections, collagen diseases and tissue damage including burns and post-operative state.
   Nephrotic syndrome.
   Pregnancy.
L. Cachexia, liver failure, many haematological disorders including leukaemia.
   Haemorrhagic conditions.
   Congenital afibrinogenaemia.
   Certain obstetric catastrophies.

PYRUVATE (SPECIAL COLLECTION)
N.R. 0·5–1·0 mg/100 ml.
R. Abnormally raised pyruvate tolerance test in vitamin B_1 deficiency.
   Congestive cardiac failure.
   Pernicious anaemia.
   Intoxication with heavy metals.
   Diabetes mellitus.

SUGAR (B—FLUORIDE BOTTLE)
N.R. 50–110 mg/100 ml.
   (True glucose levels are slightly lower.)
R. Diabetes mellitus.
   Hyperthyroidism.
   Cushing's syndrome.
   Phaeochromocytoma.
   Brain damage including subarachnoid haemorrhage.
L. Insulinoma.
   Reactive hypoglycaemia.

UREA (B)
N.R. 20–40 mg/100 ml.
R. Acute and chronic kidney disease (renal uraemia).
   Severe dehydration and circulatory collapse (pre-renal uraemia).
   Obstruction of ureter, bladder, urethra, e.g. renal calculus, carcinoma of bladder (post-renal uraemia).
L. Prolonged malnutrition and advanced liver disease.

URIC ACID (S)
N.R. 2·0–6·5 mg/100 ml.
R. Asymptomatic gout and gouty arthritis.
   Myeloid leukaemia.
   Polycythremia.
   Lesch-Nyhan syndrome.

L. Xanthinuria.
   Congenital renal tubular defects.
   Wilson's disease.

VITAMIN B$_{12}$ (S)
N.R. 190–950 μg/ml (lact. Leichmanii). —7 $N\mu g\backslash m\mathcal{l}$.
R. Many forms of acute and chronic liver disease.
   Chronic myeloid leukaemia.
   Polycythaemia vera.
   Vitamin B$_{12}$ drug therapy.

L. Pernicious anaemia.
   Malabsorption syndromes.
   Post gastrectomy syndromes.
   Surgical resection of distal ileum.

HAEMATOLOGY

HAEMOGLOBIN
N.R. depends on sex and age. *Adult males:* 14·0–18·0 g/100 ml. *Adult females:*
12·0–16·0 g/100 ml.
   In the first few days of life haemoglobin levels are higher than for
adults (14·5–24·5 g/100 ml) on the first day of life. Following this they
progressively fall to reach their lowest values at 1 year of age (11·2
g/100 ml). From this point the haemoglobin rises slowly until adult
values are reached.
R. Dehydration.
   Polycythaemia: primary (polycythaemia rubra vera)
                  secondary (e.g. the newborn, congenital heart
                           diseases, living at high altitudes).

L. Anaemias of all types.

PACKED CELL VOLUME (P.C.V.) (Haematocrit)
N.R. As with the haemoglobin this depends on the sex and age. *Adult males:*
40–54 per cent. *Adult females:* 37–47 per cent.
   As in the cases of haemoglobin levels, the values are higher in the

first few days of life (44–64 per cent on the first day of life). Following this the levels progressively fall until they reach their lowest at 1 year of age (35 per cent). They then slowly rise until adult values are reached.

R. Dehydration.

   Polycythaemia: primary (polycthaemia rubra vera)

                 secondary (e.g. the new born, congenital heart disease, pulmonary disease, living at high altitudes).

L. Anaemias of all types.

RED BLOOD CELLS

N.R. Depends on sex and age. *Adult males:* 4·6–6·2 million/cmm. *Adult females:* 4·2–5·4 million/cmm.

R. Dehydration.

   Polycythaemia: primary (polycthaemic rubra vera)

                 secondary (e.g. the newborn, congenital heart disease, pulmonary disease, living at high altitudes).

L. Anaemias of all types.

MEAN CORPUSCULAR VOLUME (M.C.V.)

N.R. 76–96 c μ.

R. Megaloblastic anaemias (anaemias due to vitamin B_{12} and or folic acid deficiency) e.g. pernicious anaemia, and malabsorption syndromes.

At birth the red cells are normally macrocytic (i.e. have a high M.C.V.). They show a progressive fall in M.C.V. over the first few weeks of life.

L. Iron deficiency anaemia.

MEAN CORPUSCULAR HAEMOGLOBIN (M.C.H.)

N.R. 27–32 μμg.

R. Macrocytic anaemias (even up to 40–50 μμg).

L. Microcytic anaemias (in iron deficiency may fall to 15 μμg).

MEAN CORPUSCULAR HAEMOGLOBIN CONCENTRATION (M.C.H.C.)

N.R. 32–36 per cent (i.e. 32–36 g haemoglobin/100 ml of packed red cells).

L. Iron deficiency anaemia.

   Overhydration.

WHITE CELL COUNT (LEUCOCYTE COUNT)

N.R. This depends on age. *Adults:* 4,000–11,000/cmm.

For the first 2 or 3 days after birth much higher levels are often found, e.g. up to 22,000/cmm.

R. Bacterial infections

leukaemias (chronic myeloid and chronic lymphatic, and some of the acute leukaemias such as acute myeloblastic and acute lymphoblastic).

L. Some viral infections

Agranulocytosis.

Some of the acute leukaemis (aleukaemic leukaemias).

Aplastic anaemia.

DIFFERENTIAL WHITE-CELL COUNT

N.R. *Adults.*

Neutrophils		
(polymorphonuclear leucocytes)	50–75%	3,000–6,000/cmm
Lymphocytes	20–45%	1,500–3,000/cmm
Monocytes	2– 6%	200– 500/cmm
Eosinophils	1– 5%	40– 440/cmm
Basophils	up to 1%	15– 100/cmm

PLATELETS (THROMBOCYTES)

N.R. 140,000–340,000/cmm.

R. Generalized infections (up to 500,000/cmm).

Surgical operations (up to twice the normal value, and the maximum rise is at the 7th to 10th post-operative day).

Thrombocythaemia (up to 2 million/cmm or more).

Post-splenectomy (the level may rise quickly after a few hours and reaches a peak at 7–10 days. Following this there is a fall to normal values over several weeks or months, although in 30 per cent of cases the platelet level will remain high permanently).

L. (Thrombocytopenia).

(1) Idiopathic.

(2) Secondary to drugs, leukaemias, aplastic anaemia and bone marrow infiltration.

ERYTHROCYTE SEDIMENTATION RATE (E.S.R.)

N.R. (Westergren's method). *Males:* 3–5 mm in 1 hour. *Females:* 4–7 mm in 1 hour.

R. Very high values are found in

Myelomatosis.

Collagen diseases such as disseminated lupus erythematosus, polyarteritis nodosa, temporal arteritis, scleroderma, dermatomyositis, and rheumatoid arthritis.

Some patients with carcinomatosis.

Cryoglobulinaemia (if the test is performed at 37°C—see below).

Macroglobulinaemia.

L. Polycythaemia.

Cryoglobulinaemia. The proteins known as cryoglobulins are, as the name suggests, precipitated in the cold, and hence when the blood is cooled down outside the body the proteins which are precipitated lead to increased viscosity which in turn prevents the red cells from settling. Hence the low sedimentation rate when the test is performed at room temperature. If, however, the blood is kept at 37°C and the test also performed at the same temperature, the E.S.R. will be very high.

RETICULOCYTES

N.R. *Adults:* 0·5–1·5 per cent.

R. Haemorrhage.

Haemolysis.

B_{12} treatment of pernicious anaemia.

Vitamin treatment of iron deficiency anaemia.

RED CELL MASS

N.R. ♂ 26–33 ml/kg.   ♀ 22–29 ml/kg.

R. Polycythaemia rubra vera.

L. All anaemias.

TOTAL PLASMA VOLUME

N.R. 40–50 ml/kg body weight.

R. Pregnancy.

Inappropriate secretion of antidiuretic hormone.

L. Dehydration (e.g. severe vomiting and diarrhoea).

BLEEDING TIME

N.R. Depends on method of examination. Up to 7 minutes.

R. Thrombocytopenia.

Severe liver disease.

Severe deficiency of certain clotting factors including fibrinogen, prothrombin, antihaemophiliac globulin (A.H.G.).

Von Willebrand's disease.

CLOTTING TIME
N.R. Depends on method of examination. 3–11 minutes.
R. Haemophilia.
    Christmas disease.
    Fibrinogen deficiency and some other clotting factor deficiencies.

PROTHROMBIN TIME (1 stage method of Quick)
N.R. Depends on laboratory technique and reagents. 12–18 seconds. The time quoted must always be compared with that of a normal control examined by the same technique on the same day.
R. Liver disease.
    Treatment with anticoagulant drugs.
    When treating a patient with anticoagulant drugs the ratio:

$$\frac{\text{patients prothrombin time (seconds)}}{\text{normal control prothrombin time (seconds)}} \text{ should range from 2–2·5.}$$

Sometimes the PROTHROMBIN INDEX is used and is determined as follows:

$$\frac{\text{normal control prothrombin time (seconds)}}{\text{patient's prothrombin time (seconds)}} \times 100\%.$$

PARTIAL THROMBOPLASTIN TIME (P.T.T.)
N.R. 45–75 seconds.
R. All coagulation defects except factor 7 deficiency.

BONE MARROW
    Examination of the bone marrow is of value in the following conditions:
1. Pernicious anaemia.
2. Other causes of vitamin B_{12} and folate deficiency.
3. Leukaemias.
4. Secondary carcinomatosis.
5. Myelomatosis.
6. Thrombocytopenia.
7. Lipid storage diseases.
8. Agranulocytosis.
9. Aplastic anaemia.
10. Myelosclerosis.

GLUCOSE-6-PHOSPHATE DEHYDROGENASE IN RED CELLS
R. Not clinically important.
L. Certain haemolytic anaemias.

URINE

δ-AMINOLAEVULINIC ACID
N.R. 0·01–0·57 mg/100 ml.
R. Acute intermittent porphyria (increased excretion may occur between acute attacks.)
   Lead intoxication.

L. Not clinically important.

CALCIUM
N.R. ♂ 100–300 mg/24 hr.   ♀ 100–250 mg/24 hr.
R. Hyperparathyroidism.
   Idiopathic hypercalciuria.
   Prolonged immobilization in bed.

L. Rickets.
   Osteomalacia.
   Hypoparathyroidism.
   Pseudohypoparathyroidism.
   Malabsorption syndromes.

CATECHOLAMINES
N.R. 240 μg/24 hr expressed as adrenaline.
R. Phaeochromocytoma.
   Neuroblastoma.
   Carcinoidosis.

L. Not clinically important.

COPPER
N.R. <50 μg/24 hr.
R. Wilson's disease (increases after penicillamine therapy).
   Conditions associated with proteinuria.

L. Not clinically important.

CREATINE
N.R. 0–50 mg/24 hr (adults).
R. Wasting muscle diseases and other conditions in which there is tissue destruction (e.g. burns, carcinomatosis).
   Hyperthyroidism.

L. Hypothyroidism.

CREATININE
N.R. *Adults:* ♂ 1·5–2·0 g/24 hr.   ♀ 0·8–1·5 g/24 hr.
R. Hypothyroidism.
   Acromegaly and gigantism.

L. Hyperthyroidism.
    Muscle wasting diseases.

ELECTROLYTES
Potassium
N.R. 35–90 mEq/24 hr.
R. High potassium intake.
    Cushing's syndrome.
    Hyperaldosteronism.
    Cortisone and ACTH therapy.
    Following use of diuretic drugs.
    Congenital renal tubular defects.
    Diuretic phase of acute tubular necrosis.
    Potassium losing nephritis.

L. Low potassium intake (particularly while on I.V. fluid therapy).
    Addison's disease.
    Pituitary insufficiency.
    Acute renal failure.

Sodium
N.R. 80–200 mEq/24 hr.
R. High salt intake.
    Addison's disease.
    Pituitary insufficiency.
    Inappropriate secretion of A.D.H.

L. Low salt intake.
    Cushing's syndrome.
    Cortisone and ACTH drug therapy.
    Hyperaldosteronism.

GONADOTROPHINS
N.R. Consult laboratory carrying out assay.
R. Throughout pregnancy (commences to rise early in pregnancy).
    During and for some years after the menopause.
    Chorion carcinoma and hydatidiform mole.
    Primary ovarian and testicular failure.

L. Ovarian and testicular failure secondary to pituitary insufficiency.
    Severe malnutrition and cachectic states.

5-HYDROXYINDOLEACETIC ACID (5HIAA)
(Patient should be on Banana free diet)
N.R. <15 mg/24 hr.

R. Carcinoid syndrome due to carcinoid **tumour** or oat celled carcinoma of lung.
Phaeochromocytoma.

L. Not clinically important.

LEAD
Accepted range. *Adults:* <80 μgm/24 hr.
R. Exposure to lead containing compounds. Further increase follows penicillamine treatment.

OESTROGENS
N.R. ♂ 10–25 μgm/24 hr.
   ♀ 5–25 μgm/24 hr at onset of menstruation.
   30–80 μgm/24 hr at ovulation.
   3–10 μgm/24 hr postmenopausal.
R. Pregnancy.
Ovarian or uterine carcinoma.
Some tumours of adrenal cortex.
Some tumours of testis.
Advanced liver disease.

L. Primary ovarian and testicular failure.
Pituitary insufficiency.

OSMOLALITY
N.R. 40–1,200 mOsmols/kg.
R. Levels must be interpreted in relation to blood osmolality. High urine osmolalities are found in dehydration when urine is concentrated and in diabetes mellitus when there is sugar in the urine.
Inappropriate secretion of A.D.H.

L. Low levels are found in water intoxication and diabetes insipidus.

17-HYDROXYCORTICOSTEROIDS
N.R. Depends on age. *Adults:* ♂ 8·0–22·0 mg/24 hr.   ♀ 4·6–17·0 mg/24 hr.
R. Cushing's syndrome (adrenocortical hyperplasia, adenoma, carcinoma of adrenal cortex, carcinoma of lung, basophil adenoma of pituitary).
Advanced liver disease.
Pregnancy.
Adrenogenital syndrome.

L. Addison's disease.
Pituitary insufficiency.

17-OXOGENIC STEROIDS (17-KETOGENIC STEROIDS)
(Very similar to 17-hydroxycorticosteroids).
N.R. Depends on age. *Adults:* ♂ 8–20 mg/24 hr.   ♀ 6–18 mg/24 hr.
R. Cushing's syndrome.
    Adrenogenital syndrome.
    A.C.T.H. treatment.
    Pregnancy.

L. Addison's disease.
    Pituitary insufficiency.
    Hypothyroidism.
    Treatment with tranquillizer drugs.

17-OXOSTEROIDS (17-KETOSTEROIDS)
N.R. Depends on age. *Adults:* ♂ 9–24 mg/24 hr.   ♀ 5–17 mg/24 hr.
R. Cushing's syndrome.
    Adrenogenital syndrome.
    A.C.T.H. treatment.
    Some ovarian tumours.
    Pregnancy.

L. Addison's disease.
    Pituitary insufficiency.
    Primary hypogonadism.
    Hypothyroidism.
    Treatment with tranquillizer drugs.

pH
N.R. 4·5–7·8.
R. Metabolic and respiratory alkalosis and renal tubular acidosis.

L. Metabolic and respiratory acidosis except for renal tubular
    acidosis.

PORPHOBILINOGEN
N.R. Up to 0·2 mg/100 ml.
R. Acute porphyria.
    Chronic liver disease.
    Following the use of certain drugs.

PORPHYRINS
Coproporphyrin N.R. 60–280 μgm/24 hr.
Uroporphyrin   N.R. 5–30 μgm/24 hr.
R. Porphyrins are raised in many forms of porphyria and lead
    intoxication.

L. Not clinically important.

PREGNANETRIOL
N.R. *Adults:* ♂ 0·4–2·4 mg/24 hr.   ♀ 0·1–3·0 mg/24 hr.
R. Adrenogenital syndrome.

L. Over treatment of adrenogenital syndrome with cortisone.

SPECIFIC GRAVITY
N.R. 1·002–1·032.
R. High levels are found with the concentrated urine of patients suffering from dehydration and in patients with diabetes mellitus with sugar in the urine; also in conditions in which there is inappropriate secretion of A.D.H.; also in any condition associated with proteinuria.

L. Low values are found with water intoxication and diabetes insipidus.

UREA
N.R. 16–35 G/24 hr. Depends on dietary protein intake.
R. High protein intake including casilan/complan.
Hyperthyroidism.
Metabolic response to trauma (including post-operative state).

L. Renal failure.
Advanced liver disease.

URIC ACID
N.R. 0·1–1·0 G/24 hr.
R. High dietary purine intake.
Myeloid leukaemia.
Polycythaemia.
Uricosuric drugs.

L. Xanthinuria.

UROBILINOGEN
N.R. <2·0 mg/24 hr.
R. Haemolytic anaemia.
Tissue haemorrhage.
Liver disease with incomplete biliary obstruction.

L. Obstructive jaundice when the biliary obstruction is complete.

4-HYDROXY-3-METHOXYMANDELIC ACID. HMMA. (V.M.A.)
N.R. 1·8–7·1 mg/24 hr.
R. Phaeochromocytoma.
Carcinoidosis.

L. Not clinically important.

CEREBROSPINAL FLUID (C.S.F.)

The cerebrospinal fluid is normally collected by the lumbar route with the patient lying horizontal on one side. The pressure is measured and fluid collected into at least two clean dry sterile containers, and sent to the laboratory at once. When an assay for sugar is required additional C.S.F. must be collected into a fluoride bottle. If blood is present and equally mixed in both containers it suggests a diagnosis of subarachnoid haemorrhage, while if it is present in greater excess in the first bottle than in the second the cause is more likely to have been a 'traumatic tap' at lumbar puncture.

Pressure 70–180 mm water.

Appearance Absolutely clear.

After centrifugation the supernatant can be inspected. If clear this confirms that blood has been recently mixed with the C.S.F. A yellowish colour (xanthochromia) indicates that the cells have been in contact with the C.S.F. for 48 hours or more. The presence of a small fibrin clot suggests a high protein content. Cloudiness indicates the presence of red or white cells.

Cells 0–5 lymphocytes/cmm.

PROTEIN

In the lumbar C.S.F. an average of up to 40 mg/100 ml is normal but in many subjects this rises slowly with age up to 60 mg/100 ml in the seventh decade.

PANDY TEST FOR EXCESS GLOBULIN

This is always positive in the presence of a high total C.S.F. protein. A positive test therefore only assumes significance if the total protein is normal and suggests a diagnosis of demyelinating disease (e.g. multiple sclerosis) or syphilis.

The γ globulin content of C.S.F. is usually about 10 per cent of the total protein content.

(In C.S.F. obtained directly from the cerebral ventricles the protein content is much lower, normal levels being 5–10 mg/100 ml.)

The causes of raised total protein are numerous, and the diagnostic value lies more in the finding of a normal concentration, which *excludes* many conditions.

COLLOIDAL GOLD (LANGE) TEST

This test depends upon the precipitation of a colloidal suspension of gold at different dilutions by variations in the albumin/globulin ratio and the ratios of the individual globulins.

0 = No precipitation.
5 = Complete precipitation.

0000000000	'No change' Normal	
0001110000	Normal	
0001233210	'Meningitic type'	Acute meningitis.
0123321000	'Tabetic type'	Tabes dorsalis (syphilis).
5544322110	'Paretic type'	Demyelination diseases (e.g. multiple sclerosis).
		General paralysis of insane (syphilis).
		Carcinomatous meningitis.
		Subacute inclusion body encephalitis.

SUGAR
N.R. 50–80 mg/100 ml.
If values outside this range are obtained the blood sugar level should be checked. In the presence of a normal blood sugar a low C.S.F. sugar is found in bacterial carcinomatous and tuberculous meningitis, though in all these cases a low C.S.F. sugar is a late manifestation. A value within the normal range should not be regarded as evidence against the diagnosis of one of these conditions.

CHLORIDE
This assay is of no practical clinical value.

Function, tolerance, clearance tests

TESTS OF CARBOHYDRATE METABOLISM

Glucose tolerance test
N.R. Fasting blood sugar 50–110 mg/100 ml. Peak value 180 mg/100 ml.
Fasting level should be regained by 120 minutes.
No sugar should appear in the urine.

Increased tolerance
Anterior pituitary insufficiency and malabsorption syndromes.

Decreased tolerance
The most important cause is diabetes mellitus but other conditions include thyrotoxicosis, Cushing's syndrome, some post-gastrectomy patients (lag curve), and conditions in which there is 'tissue damage' including cardiac infarction, extensive burns and subarachnoid haemorrhage.

The patient should be on a diet containing at least 300 grams carbohydrate for 3 days prior to the test.

50 G glucose is given orally in the morning to the fasting patient.

Venous blood is collected before the glucose load and at 30, 60, 90 and 120 minutes and urine at 60 and 120 minutes.

Cortisone glucose tolerance test

N.R. As for glucose tolerance test.

Decreased tolerance is indicative of 'pre diabetes'. The test is similar to the glucose tolerance test except that the patient is given 50–62·5 mg cortisone orally $8\frac{1}{2}$ and 2 hours before the glucose load.

Pyruvate metabolism test

N.R. Fasting blood pyruvate up to 1·0 mg/100 ml.
      60 minute sample   up to 1·3 mg/100 ml.
      90 minute sample   up to 1·3 mg/100 ml.

A normal fasting pyruvate followed by an excessive and prolonged rise after glucose which reverts to normal after vitamin B_1 therapy is indicative of vitamin B_1 deficiency.

The patient is rested and fasted overnight. Two oral doses of 50 grams glucose are given at 0 and 30 minutes and blood is taken for pyruvate assay prior to the first glucose load and at 60 and 90 minutes. The blood is collected by the laboratory staff.

Tolbutamide tolerance test

N.R. Maximal fall of blood *glucose* is at 20–45 minutes. The level to which the blood glucose falls is less significant than the level at the end of 3 hours which should be at least 70 per cent of the fasting level.

Used in the diagnosis of Insulinoma.

The patient should be on a diet containing at least 300 grams carbohydrate for 3 days prior to the test. 1 gram tolbutamide is given I.V. over a two minute period to the recumbent patient fasted overnight. Blood is taken for *glucose* prior to the tolbutamide injection and afterwards at 10, 20, 30, 60, 90, 120, 150 and 180 minutes. Sometimes blood may also be taken for insulin assays. If so heparinized blood should be collected before the tolbutamide is given and at 2, 4, 6, 10, 20, 30, 60 and 90 minutes. The red cells must be separated at once as each specimen is collected and the plasma placed in the 'deep-freeze' at $-20°C$.

Intravenous glucose and hydrocortisone should be available to terminate the test quickly in the event of severe or prolonged hypoglycaemia.

Insulin tolerance test

N.R. Blood glucose should fall to 50 per cent fasting level within the first 20–30 minutes and return to the fasting level within 2 hours.

Measurements of plasma cortisol and growth hormone are sometimes also made during an insulin tolerance test.

Failure of the blood glucose to return to normal within 2 hours points to lack of pituitary reserve.

The patient should be on a diet containing at least 300 grams carbohydrate for 3 days prior to the test.

0·1 unit soluble insulin/kg body weight is given I.V. to the fasting patient and blood samples for *glucose* are collected prior to the injection of insulin and at 5, 10, 15, 20, 45, 60, 90 and 120 minutes.

This test may be dangerous in patients with pituitary insufficiency in whom an initial test using 0·03 unit/kg body weight of insulin should be tried. In all cases intravenous glucose should be available for immediate administration.

Insulin-glucose test

N.R. Fall of blood glucose to 50 per cent fasting level at 30 minutes, followed by a sharp rise at 60 minutes to between 100 and 200 mg/100 ml and then a gradual fall.

Used as a test of pituitary 'reserve function'.

Instructions for the test are as for the insulin tolerance test except that in addition 0·8 g glucose/kg body weight is given orally within the first 30 minutes of the standard I.V. dose of 0·1 unit/kg body weight of insulin.

Glucagon test

N.R. Rise of blood *glucose* of 40 mg/100 ml or more in the first $\frac{1}{2}$ hour and a peak increase over the fasting level of 30–90 mg between $\frac{1}{2}$ and 1 hour and returning to near the fasting level within 3 hours.

This test is used in the differential diagnosis of spontaneous hypoglycaemia and in the investigation of glycogen storage disease.

The patient should be on a diet containing 300 g carbohydrate for 3 days prior to the test.

1 mg glucagon is given intramuscularly to the fasting patient and blood samples are taken for *glucose* assay prior to the injection and at 15, 30 minutes and then half-hourly for 3 hours.

Ischaemic exercise lactate test

N.R. Healthy subjects show a rapid rise of blood lactate in response to ischaemic exercise followed by a more gradual fall to normal within 15 minutes.

In patients with muscle phosphorylase deficiency (McArdle's syndrome) and certain other muscle enzyme deficiencies there is no rise in blood lactate during ischaemic exercise.

The patient must fast overnight and be completely at rest in bed. A tourniquet is applied to the lower arm just above the wrist and blood samples are taken from the forearm veins without venous stasis, by the laboratory staff before and after standardized exercise of the forearm muscles. During the period of exercise a second tourniquet is applied to the upper arm to render the muscles ischaemic.

ENDOCRINE FUNCTION TESTS

Function tests of the adrenal cortex
Normal values of plasma cortisol and urine excretion of adreno-cortical steroids are given in chapter 3 p. 23, 39, 40.

Adrenocorticotrophic hormone (A.C.T.H.) stimulation test
N.R. Rise in urine 24 hr 17-hydroxycorticosteroid excretion on the third day of stimulation of at least 30 mg above the base-line excretion.

L. Addison's disease.

A base-line 24 hour urine collection is made. The patient is then given 100 units of long acting A.C.T.H. gel I.M. daily for 3 days. Further 24 hour urine collections are made for the 3 days of stimulation.

Rarely aphylactic reactions to the injection may be encountered.

Synacthen test
N.R. Base-line plasma cortisol should be not less than 6 μgm/100 ml. 30 minute plasma cortisol should be not less than 18 μgm/100 ml with a rise of not less than 7 μgm/100 ml.

This test is used in similar circumstances to the A.C.T.H. stimulation test, but the result is available much more quickly and it may be adapted for use with out-patients. 250 μgm synacthen is given intra-muscularly and blood for plasma cortisol is taken before and 30 minutes afterwards.

Single dose dexamethasone suppression test
N.R. Plasma cortisol after dexamethasone should be suppressed by at least 70 per cent to less than 6·5 μgm/100 ml.

Used to confirm the diagnosis of Cushing's syndrome in which there is a fall in plasma cortisol of less than 30 per cent in most cases and with absolute plasma cortisol levels remaining above 13 μgm/100 ml. 2 mg dexamethasone is given orally between 11.30 p.m. and midnight.

PITUITARY FUNCTION TESTS

Anterior pituitary
Direct radioimmunoassay of pituitary hormones in blood is carried out by some laboratories but these are highly specialized

procedures and are not generally available. They include assays of adrenocorticotrophic hormone, thyroid stimulating hormone, and gonadotrophins.

Growth hormone assays are however now being carried out more frequently and are of use in assessing the cause of some cases of dwarfism and delayed puberty, and in association with glucose tolerance tests in the assessment of the activity of the disease process in cases of gigantism and acromegely.

Metopirone test

N.R. An increase of approximately six-fold in the excretion over the base-line of adrenocortical steroids in the urine.

L. Indicates a fairly severe decrease in pituitary reserve function; some 80 per cent destruction of the anterior pituitary being necessary to produce a definitely positive result.

This test may predispose some subjects to collapse from cortisol deficiency, particularly in the case of children or adults undergoing surgical operations.

The dose of metopirone is 0·75 gm orally 4 hourly for 48 hours.

Pyrogen test

N.R. Marked increase in the level of plasma steroids following the I.V. administration of a bacterial pyrogen.

L. Decreased pituitary reserve function.

A bacterial pyrogen (ORGANON) is administered I.V. in a dose of 0·005 gm/kg body weight, and blood is taken for estimation of plasma steroids immediately before and 3 hours after the injection. If the patient complains of headache or muscle cramps, aspirin may be given without interfering with the test. *Intravenous hydrocortisone should be available for immediate termination of the test in the event of signs of collapse in those patients with poor pituitary reserve.*

Water excretion test

N.R. 50 per cent or more of the total volume of water taken should be excreted during the first two hours and approximately 80 per cent or more during 4 hours. The urine specific gravity should fall to 1·002 and the osmolality to less than 80 mOsmols/kg during the test.

L. Failure to dilute the urine and excrete the water load is found in the following conditions: Addison's disease, pituitary insufficiency, steatorrhoea, congestive heart failure, advanced liver disease and renal failure. If the test is repeated after oral administration of 100 mg cortisone, an improved result would point to the original diagnosis being pituitary insufficiency or primary adrenocortical failure.

The patient is fasted overnight and the bladder emptied in the morning. 20 ml/kg body weight of water is taken orally within 30 minutes and urine is collected hourly for 4 hours.

Note this test may lead to water intoxication.

POSTERIOR PITUITARY

Water deprivation and vasopressin test. See Urine concentration test. Chapter 3 p. 53.

N.R. It is not possible to give exact figures for the response to this test because the normal range is so wide. In the normal there should be a marked increase in urine osmolality to approximately 800 mOsmols/kg with water deprivation (S.G. 1·022) (see water concentration test).

L. In the absence of an osmotic diuresis failure to concentrate the urine would point to diabetes insipidus either of pituitary or renal origin, and patients would lose weight steadily with water restriction. (Not more than 4 per cent total body weight loss should be allowed as dehydration may become severe and is dangerous in these patients.) Those with pituitary diabetes insipidus will show a marked increase of urine osmolality after administration of vasopressin but there will be no response in patients with nephrogenic diabetes insipidus. The effect of vasopressin however is sometimes not marked in polyuric patients and its effect may be enhanced by restricting fluid intake before its administration.

The main differential diagnosis in a polyuric patient is psychogenic water drinking and it should be noted that the administration of vasopressin to these patients may precipitate acute water intoxication.

THYROID FUNCTION TESTS

Basal metabolic rate (B.M.R.)
N.R. ±15 per cent of normal on the Robertson and Reid standard.
R. Thyrotoxicosis, blood diseases including leukaemias and severe anaemia, and febrile conditions, malignant disease, adrenocrotical hyperfunction, pregnancy.

L. Hypothyrodism (myxoedema), pituitary insufficiency.

The patient must be absolutely basal for this investigation. Admission overnight to a separate room is necessary and the test is often repeated the following morning. Accurate measurements of the patient's height and weight are necessary.

Protein bound iodine (P.B.I.)
N.R. 4–8 μgm/100 ml.
R. Thyrotoxicosis, pregnancy, drug therapy with oestrogens (including oral contraceptives) and iodine containing compounds.

L. Hypothyroidism either primary or secondary to pituitary insufficiency. Many forms of drug therapy including steroids Nephrotic syndrome. Treatment with triiodothyronine.

Blood is taken by the laboratory staff in a special syringe and container. The patient must have had no iodine-containing medicines and preferably have been on a fish-free diet for several days before the test. Many compounds used for radiological contrast studies contain iodine and interfere with this test for months or years.

Triiodothyronine resin uptake (T_3)
N.R. 25–35 per cent.
R. Thyrotoxicosis, many drugs including hormonal preparations, anticoagulants, salicylates and phenybutazone, some liver diseases, and nephrotic syndrome.

L. Hypothyroidism either primary or secondary to pituitary insufficiency, oestrogen drug therapy, pregnancy, and some liver diseases.

No special preparation of the patient is necessary but it should be noted as indicated above that a number of drugs, particularly hormonal preparations interfere with the test.

Thyroxine Assay In a few specialized departments direct radioimmunoassay of free thyroxine (T_4) is becoming available.

Radioactive tests of thyroid function other than T_3 test
These differ from the T_3 test in that radioactive iostope is given to the patient. They are specialized procedures often carried out by departments of physics who issue their own instructions and normal values.

They consist of:

1. Thyroid uptake of radio-iodine (4 hours, 24 hours) with and without thyroid stimulating hormone (T.S.H.) stimulation and triiodothyronine (T_3) suppression.

2. Urine excretion of radioactive iodine at 24 and 48 hours.

3. Measurement of radioactive protein bound iodine in the serum.

PARATHYROID FUNCTION TESTS

Renal excretion of phosphate
Renal phosphate clearance (P.C.) N.R. 6–15 ml/minute.
Tubular reabsorption of phosphate (T.R.P.) N.R. 84 per cent–94 per cent.
Phosphate excretion index (P.E.I.) N.R. 0.0 ± 0.09.
These tests are used in the diagnosis of hyperparathyroidism and hypoparathyroidism.

	P.C.	T.R.P.	P.E.I.
Hyperparathyroidism	↑	↓	↑
Hypoparathyroidism	↓	↑	↓

Other conditions however such as vitamin D intoxication and congenital renal tubular abnormalities (e.g. De Toni-Fanconi syndrome) in which there is an abnormality in renal phosphate excretion will produce abnormal results.

The patient should fast overnight but water should be taken to ensure an adequate urine output. Two consecutive one hour urine collections are made and blood is taken at the mid-point of each. The test is combined with creatinine clearance.

Sodium phytate test for early hypoparathyroidism
N.R. No fall of serum calcium below the lower limit of normal (9·0 mg/100 ml). Patients with early hypoparathyrodism but with a serum calcium still within the limits of normal, on a normal diet, will show a fall of serum calcium below 9·0 mg/100 ml.

The patient is placed on a low calcium diet, and sodium phytate 9 G daily in divided doses *with* the main meals given for one week. The serum calcium is assayed before and during phytate administration.

Parathormone test for pseudo-hypoparathyroidism (*Elsworth-Howard test*)
The normal subject and the patient with hypoparathyroidism show a 2–3 fold increase of phosphate output in the urine. Patients with pseudo-hypoparathyroidism who are unable to respond to the hormone show no change.

The patient is placed on a low phosphate diet for 2–3 days prior to the test and should fast overnight. Water intake should be encouraged to ensure an adequate output of urine. Urine is collected hourly for 3 hours before, and for 5 hours after, an intravenous injection of 200 units fresh parathormone. Blood is sometimes collected before and after the injection for phosphate clearance studies.

A normal subject should be used as a control to check the potency of the parathormone preparation.

Cortisone test for hypercalcaemia
Cortisone 150 mg daily by mouth in divided doses may be given for 10 days as a diagnostic test to patients with a high serum calcium. In those with sarcoidosis or vitamin D intoxication there will be a significant decrease in the serum calcium but there will be no change in patients with hyperparathyroidism.

GASTRIC AND INTESTINAL FUNCTION TESTS

Augmented histamine test meal
N.R. Maximal secretion of acid occurs in period 15–30 minutes up to 11·6 mEq/min.

R. In duodenal ulcer and particularly the Zollinger-Ellison syndrome.

L. Gastric ulcer and particularly pernicious anaemia. (Absent.)

The patient fasts for 12 hours after which the whole of the resting gastric juice is aspirated, via a naso-gastric tube.

100 mg mepyramine maleate is given *intramuscularly* and the gastric juice aspirated every 5 minutes for the next 30 minutes and added to the resting sample. 30 minutes after administering the mepyramine maleate, histamine acid phosphate 0·04 mg/kg body weight to a maximum of 2·0 mg is injected *subcutaneously* and the gastric juice aspirated every 5 minutes for the next 60 minutes, being placed into four containers labelled 0–15 minutes, 15–30 minutes, 30–45 minutes, 45–60 minutes.

During the collection of specimens both the position of the tube and the patient should be changed to ensure maximal collection of gastric juice. Best results are generally obtained wtih the patient in the left lateral position.

Pentagastrin test meal
N.R. Maximal secretion occurs in the 10–30 minute period and the results calculated on this are similar to those of the augmented histamine test meal.

6 μgm/kg body weight is injected intramuscularly after an overnight fast and gastric juice is collected by continuous suction for 30 minutes in three 10 minute samples.

Faecal fat excretion
N.R. Average daily excretion of 5 G or less of faecal fatty acids.

R. Coeliac disease, sprue, pancreatic disease, infiltrative diseases of the small intestine including the reticuloses.

The patient should have been on a diet containing 50–150 G fat. (This is the fat content of an 'ordinary' hospital diet.) All stool specimens are collected with or without an oral carmine marker for at least 4 days and preferably 6 days. Sometimes chromium sesquioxide is used as a marker.

Xylose absorption test
N.R. Blood level 25–40 mg/100 ml at 90–120 minutes.
5-hour urine excretion at least 4·2 G.

R. Not clinically important.

L. Same conditions as those causing raised faecal fat excretion except for pancreatic disease.

25 GD-xylose are given orally to the patient fasted overnight. Blood is collected between 90 and 120 minutes and urine over a period of 5 hours. It is important to maintain an adequate urine flow by giving the patient water to drink (500 ml) during the test.

Vitamin A absorption test
N.R. A rise of plasma vitamin A to 500 I.U./100 ml or more is the normal response and is strong evidence for *excluding* malabsorption syndromes (see faecal fat excretion).
L. *Suggests* malabsorption syndromes.

For this test the patient should *not* fast. Blood is taken for vitamin A assay at the beginning of the test and again 5 hours after the oral ingestion of 350,000 I.U. vitamin A in arachis oil.

LIVER FUNCTION TESTS

Bilirubin
N.R. <0·8 mg/100 ml.
R. All forms of jaundice.
>   Direct positive reaction Van den Berg (conjugated) in obstructive and hepatic jaundice.
>   Indirect positive reaction Van den Bergh (unconjugated) in haemolytic jaundice.

Total Protein and Protein Fractions } See Chapter 3 p. 29.

S.G.O.T. (*Serum Glutamic-Oxalacetic Transaminase*) See Chapter 3 p. 26.

S.G.P.T. (*Serum Glutamic-Pyruvate Transaminase*) See Chapter 3 p. 26.

Alkaline Phosphatase See Chapter 3 p. 25.

Turbidity tests
Kunkel (zinc sulphate) N.R. 2–8 units.
R. Many conditions in which there is increased globulin levels in serum.
Thymol turbidity N.R. 0–4 units.

R. Some conditions in which there is increased globulin levels in serum but particularly in the *active* phase of hepatitis.

(Bromsulphthalein)B.S.P. excretion
5 mg/kg body weight B.S.P. is injected I.V. in a 5 per cent solution, with the patient fasting. Venous blood is withdrawn at 5 and 45 minutes.
N.R. <5 per cent B.S.P. remaining at 45 minutes.
   A sensitive test of liver function in the absence of jaundice.

RENAL FUNCTION TESTS

Blood Urea. See p. 31.

Blood Creatinine. See p. 23.

Urea Clearance
N.R. Maximal clearance 75 ml/min. is 100 per cent. Normal Range 85–130 per cent. Standard clearance 54 ml/min. is 100 per cent. Normal Range 75–120 per cent.
L. Renal glomerular failure due to many forms of renal disease, e.g.
      chronic nephritis, chronic pyelonephritis.
     Circulatory failure.

Ideally the patient should fast overnight but water intake should be encouraged to ensure an adequate urine output not only to aid the collection of specimens but to achieve a urine flow of greater than 2 ml/min. Under these conditions the maximal clearance can be calculated. This is more satisfactory than the standard clearance. In children a correction must be made for the body surface area.

Creatinine clearance (Endogenous, i.e. oral creatinine not administered)
N.R. 112 ± 15 ml/minute.
L. Renal glomerular failure due to many forms of renal disease, e.g.
      chronic nephritis, chronic pyelonephritis.
     Circulatory failure.

Ideally the patient should fast overnight, but water should be taken to ensure adequate urine output. Two consecutive 1 hour urine collections are made and blood is taken at the mid-point of each. This test may be combined with renal phosphate excretion tests. Sometimes a whole 24-hour urine collection is made and blood taken once during this period.

Urine concentration test. See Water deprivation and vasopressin test.
   Chapter 3 p. 48.
N.R. In at least one specimen of urine the specific gravity should be greater than 1·022 or the osmolality greater than 800 mOsmols/kg.
L. Lower results than this in the absence of diabetes insipidus
   suggest impaired tubular function.

All fluids are witheld from 8 a.m. and the bladder emptied at 8 p.m. Urine is collected as passed until 8 a.m. the following morning. The specific gravity and osmolality of all specimens during the second 12-hour period are measured.

More specialized tests of renal function —normal values
Renal plasma flow 612 ± 68 ml/minute.
Maximal glucose reabsorption capacity T.M.G. 323 ± 64 mg/minute.
Maximal para-aminohippuric acid excretory capacity Tm.P.A.H. 68 ± 11
  mg/minute.

FUNCTION TESTS OF VITAMIN DEFICIENCY

Vitamin A Absorption Test. p. 52.

Vitamin B_{12} absorption test (Schilling test—modified)
N.R. Urine radioactivity 10·5–25·7 per cent of administered dose in 24 hours.
R. Not clinically important.

L. Pernicious anaemia and malabsorption syndromes. In patients
  with pernicious anaemia normal response occurs in part 2. In
  patients with malabsorption syndromes there is an abnormal
  response in parts 1 and 2 but normal in part 3 (see below), if the
  malabsorption is due to the presence of bacteria in the gut.

Part 1. The patient is fasted overnight, but is allowed to drink water. An oral dose of 0·5 μg (approximately 0·5 μc) ^{57}Co labelled vitamin B_{12} is administered together with 1,000 μg of stable vitamin vitamin B_{12} intramuscularly, and the fast continued for a further 2 hours. A 24 hour sample of urine is collected as from administration of vitamin B_{12}, and blood for serum radioactivity assay at 8 hours.

Part 2. The test is repeated, as for part 1, but in addition the patient receives a capsule containing intrinsic factor with the oral dose of ^{57}Co vitamin B_{12}.

Part 3. As for part 2, except that the patient is treated with tetra-cycline 500 mg 6–8 hourly orally for at least 5 days prior to, and during the test.

Red cell transketolase activity
This enzyme is normally found in red and white blood cells. Its activity is much reduced by vitamin B_1 deficiency for which it may be a sensitive and specific test, particularly when there is an increased activity following the addition of thiamine pyrophosphate to the test system. Heparinized blood is collected together with an additional sample in sequestrene for P.C.V.

Tryptophan load test for vitamin B_6 deficiency

N.R. 1–3 mg xanthurenic acid/24 hours is excreted in the urine following the tryptophan load

Patients with vitamin B_6 deficiency may excrete up to 60 mg/24 hours after trytophan load.

24 hour urine collections are made before and after an oral dose of 2 G L-trytophan, and preserved with 25 ml normal hydrochloric acid. The urine is analysed for xanthurenic acid.

Vitamin C saturation test

N.R. At least 50 mg ascorbic acid (vitamin C) will be found in the 2 hour urine sample on the first or second day.

Used to confirm a suspected diagnosis of scurvy or vitamin C deficiency. Ascorbic acid 70 mg/*stone* body weight is given daily by mouth at 10 a.m. A two hour urine collection is made between four and six hours later in a dark container with 20 ml glacial acetic acid and *sent at once for analysis.*

4

Disorders in which investigations play an important part in diagnosis and treatment

In this chapter tests are grouped according to the patient's clinical diagnosis. Thus if a patient is suspected of suffering from, say, diabetic coma, all the biochemical investigations of diagnostic importance are listed under this heading. This chapter should be particularly useful in indicating further tests that are likely to be required.

Alimentary system, liver and pancreas

Duodenal ulcer

Augmented histamine test meal shows high gastric acidity, both basal and following histamine stimulation. High acidity after pentagastrin.

Faecal occult blood test may be positive.

Gastric ulcer

Blood and mucus may be present in gastric aspirate and occult blood in stools.

Free and total gastric acid may vary within wide limits but on the whole tend to be subnormal.

Gastric carcinoma

Blood and mucus in test meal samples. No free acid and reduced total acid following histamine stimulation, or pentagastrin

Test for occult blood in stools often positive.

Pyloric stenosis

Aspiration of gastric contents shows large volumes containing undigested food, but no bile pigments.

If associated with vomiting there will be the features of dehydration, sodium and chloride deficiency and to a lesser extent potassium deficiency. Metabolic alkalosis.

Ulcerative colitis and watery diarrhoea

Blood and mucus in stools. Iron deficiency anaemia. Dehydration, sodium and potassium depletion. In later stages decreased total protein in plasma with decrease in albumin/globulin ratio. Metabolic acidosis.

Post-gastrectomy syndrome

Low serum vitamin B_{12}.

Glucose tolerance test shows 'lag curve', followed by reactive hypoglycaemia.

Steatorrhea may be present.

Low serum iron.

Idiopathic steatorrhea

Increased faecal fat and faecal nitrogen.

Macrocytic anaemia. Low blood folate. Abnormal formimino-glutamic acid (F.I.G.L.U.) excretion. Low blood vitamin B_{12}. Schilling test shows poor, but not absence of, vitamin B_{12} absorption, unaffected by intrinsic factor. Low serum iron. Low serum calcium and phosphate. Raised serum alkaline phosphatase. Low urine calcium.

Vitamin A absorption test abnormal. Abnormal xylose absorption. Dehydration, sodium and potassium depletion. Increased glucose tolerance. Decreased plasma proteins with decreased albumin/globulin ratio.

Liver cell failure

INCREASE OF: blood ammonia, blood and urine amino acids, serum bilirubin, alkaline phosphatase, S.G.O.T., lactic dehydrogenase, aldolase. Urine porphyrins slightly raised.

DECREASE OF: Serum albumin, albumin/globulin ratio blood urea.

Failure of normal rise in blood sugar following injection of adrenaline and of glucagon.

Glucose Tolerance. Low fasting blood sugar may be present—lag curve with reactive hypoglycaemia later.

Galactose Tolerance abnormal.

Bromsulphthalein excretion test abnormal.

Infective hepatitis

BEFORE CLINICAL JAUNDICE: Bilirubin appears in the urine. B.S.P. test abnormal.

AFTER ONSET OF CLINICAL JAUNDICE: Serum bilirubin rises. Positive direct Van den Bergh reaction. Decrease in serum albumin, with increase in serum globulins.

Increase of Thymol turbidity and Kunkel turbidity tests.

Rise in both S.G.O.T. and S.G.P.T. but with a fall in S.G.O.T./ S.G.P.T. ratio. Raised I.C.D.

Slight rise in urine porphyrins.

Cirrhosis of liver

Decrease in serum albumin with increase in globulins.

Kunkel turbidity raised.

Serum alkaline phosphatase may be raised.

Galactose tolerance test abnormal.

S.G.O.T. raised. Urine porphyrins slightly raised.

Abnormal B.S.P. test.

Primary biliary cirrhosis

Very high serum cholesterol and total serum lipids.

Raised serum bilirubin (conjugated) and alkaline phosphatase.

Bilirubin present in urine. Decreased faecal pigments. Steatorrhoea.

Secondary carcinoma of the liver

Serum bilirubin may be normal or raised (conjugated). Bilirubin is often present in urine.

Raised alkaline phosphatase and raised serum 5-nucleotidase.

Raised S.G.O.T.   I.C.D.

Abnormal B.S.P. test.

Extra hepatic biliary obstruction

Very high serum bilirubin (conjugated) with positive direct Van den Bergh reaction.

High bilirubin content in urine.

Very high serum alkaline phosphatase. S.G.O.T. and S.G.P.T. also raised.

Serum cholesterol raised.

When obstruction is complete urobilin disappears from urine and faeces. Steatorrhoea.

Familial hyperbilirubinaemia

Several forms of familial hyperbilirubinaemia exist. Those which survive early childhood are benign conditions in which all tests of liver function are normal apart from the presence of a slight or moderately raised serum bilirubin. The two commoner forms are the Gilbert type in which the direct Van den Bergh reaction is negative and bilirubin absent from the urine, and the Dubin-Johnson type in which the direct Van den Bergh reaction is positive, and bile is present in the urine.

Acute pancreatitis

Marked rise in both serum and urine amylase. Also transient rise in serum lipase.

Obstruction of pancreatic duct

Steatorrhoea but xylose tolerance test normal.
Reduced amylase, lipase and trypsin in duodenal juice.
Increase of faecal nitrogen.

Carcinoma of pancreas

Often biliary obstruction is present with the associated biochemical changes (vide supra.)

Cystic fibrosis of pancreas

High sodium chloride content of sweat and saliva.
Malabsorption syndrome with increased faecal fat.
Xylose absorption normal.
Duodenal and faecal trypsin activity reduced.
Duodenal juice contains a mucoprotein which is rendered insoluble in water by adding a 1 : 1 mixture of benzene and ethyl alcohol.

Islet cell tumour (insulinoma)

Fasting blood sugar low and may become very low with prolonged fast.
Prolonged glucose tolerance test shows a 'flat' curve with low glucose levels towards the end.
Tolbutamide tolerance test produces marked and prolonged hypoglycaemia.
Glucagon test produces a transient rise in blood glucose followed by prolonged hypoglycaemia.

Diabetes mellitus

Fasting blood sugar high with glycosuria.

Decreased glucose tolerance. May be normal in 'pre-diabetes' in which case becomes abnormal after cortisone.

Serum chlesterol raised.

Pyruvate metabolism test abnormal.

Diabetic coma (ketosis)

Blood sugar high or very high, together with glycosuria and large urine output. Urine pale but osmolality and specific gravity high.

Ketones in blood and urine.

Metabolic acidosis with low blood pH and alkali reserve, and low urine pH. Low $paCO_2$.

Raised plasma inorganic phosphate.

High plasma sodium and potassium, though both may fall rapidly with treatment.

Very high plasma osmolality. Raised blood urea.

Blood diseases

THE ANAEMIAS

The cells found in the peripheral blood are formed in the bone marrow. In adults the main sites of formation are the proximal ends of long bones, the vertebrae, ribs, skull, pelvis and clavicles. In the foetus, islands of blood forming tissue are present in the liver and spleen. A regression to this more primitive state is found in certain diseases in adults where the bone marrow is unable to function, in which case islands of bone marrow cells appear again in the liver and spleen (myeloid metaplasia).

A classification of anaemia follows:

A. *Impairment of formation of red cells*
1. Deficiency of essential substances necessary for blood formation, e.g. iron, vitamin B_{12} folic acid, vitamin C, protein and copper.
2. Abnormality of the bone marrow cells which are unable to function normally (e.g. leukaemia).
3. Infiltration or replacement of marrow with abnormal tissue (e.g. carcinomatosis, myelofibrosis).
4. Toxic effects of substances accumulating in the body in certain conditions (e.g. uraemia, chronic infections).
5. Toxic effects of drugs and poisons on the bone marrow, e.g. benzene.

B. *Loss of, or destruction of blood*
1. Haemorrhage (e.g. gastrointestinal).
2. Haemolysis (*red cell defects* such as congenital spherocytic haemolytic anaemia and haemoglobin abnormalities sich as sickle cell anaemia and other haemoglobinopathies; also *extracorpuscular factors* such as autoantibodies, certain drugs, certain vegetables, snake venoms, and some infections such as malaria). In addition certain diseases such as collagen diseases, lymphomas and leukaemias, and cirrhosis of the liver, may be accompanied by some degree of haemolysis.

Iron deficiency anaemia
Haemoglobin low.
Blood film shows anisocytosis, poikilocytosis, and hypochromia of the red cells.
Serum iron low.
Marrow—stainable iron very low.

Causes of iron deficiency anaemia
The commonest type of anaemia usually seen in young women is due to iron deficiency, the causes of which are:

1. Insufficient iron intake in the food.
2. Normal iron intake but deficient absorption. e.g. Malabsorption Syndrome
3. Normal intake and absorption, but loss of blood (e.g. excess menstrual loss or gastrointestinal bleeding—visible occult.)

Pernicious anaemia
Haemoglobin will be low in advanced cases (even down to 3 G/100 ml, i.e. 20 per cent in very severe cases). Macrocytes are seen in the peripheral blood film even in early cases when haemoglobin level may be little affected. White cells and platelets are reduced slightly in many patients.
Serum vitamin B_{12} level is low (less than 180 $\mu\mu$g/ml, and usually ess than 100 $\mu\mu$g/ml) as long as the patient has not received vitamin B_{12} injections previously.
No free hydrochloric acid can be demonstrated in the gastric juice, even after histamine or pentagastrin stimulation.
The bone marrow is megaloblastic.

The Schilling test shows very low absorption of ^{57}Co vitamin B$_{12}$ (less than 3 per cent) in part 1. Part 2, with instrinsic factor, will show increased absorption.

Several days after the Schilling test, in which 1,000 μg of vitamin B$_{12}$ is given, the peripheral blood reticulocytes will rise, the height depending mainly on the severity of the anaemia.

Serum Lactate Dehydrogenase raised.

Anaemias related to pregnancy

1. *Physiological anaemia* is the commonest type of anaemia of pregnancy commencing about the 8th week and increasing progressively until the 30th week when haemoglobin levels of 11·0 G/100 ml are typical. It is known that

(*a*) Plasma volume progressively rises (by 30–40 per cent) and that

(*b*) Red cell mass increases in pregnancy (by 15 per cent) although the latter does in fact show a slight fall in the early weeks of pregnancy.

The disparity between the two, results in haemodilution and the overall effect is that the haemoglobin level decreases.

2. *Iron deficiency anaemia* may occur in pregnancy. Typical haemoglobin levels would be less than 10·0 G/100 ml.

3. *Folate deficiency* may lead to megaloblastic anaemia of pregnancy, and is probably due to utilization of this vitamin by the foetus leads to deprivation of the mother.

4. *Any other anaemia* associated by chance with pregnancy.

5. *Post partum* anaemia—due to blood loss at parturition.

Physiological blood changes in pregnancy

Haemoglobin—decreases

P.C.V.—decreases

E.S.R.—increased (mainly in the 3rd trimester).

White cells may show slight increase.

Haemolytic anaemias

Normal red cells have a life of about 120 days. This may be considerably shortened in haemolytic anaemias. There are two major types:

1. *Intracorpuscular defects:* the defect lies in the red cell itself e.g. hereditary spherocytosis (acholuric jaundice) haemoglobinopathies and non-spherocytic congenital haemolytic anaemia.

2. *Extracorpuscular defects:* the defect lies in the plasma and secondarily affects the red cells (e.g. haemolytic disease of the new born, haemolysis due to chemical agents, acquired haemolytic anaemia, and haemolytic anaemia in severe infections).

Raised serum bilirubin (1–3 mg/100 ml or occasionally higher) indirect Van den Bergh

Faecal Stercobilinogen increased (up to 1,000 mg/day, normal levels being 50–300 mg).

Urine urobilinogen increased in acute haemolytic anaemia.

Serum haptoglobins: decreased in haemolytic disease (less than 10 mg/100 ml. Normal level = 20–200 mg/100 ml).

Haemoglobinaemia may be present in acute Haemolytic anaemias.

Haemoglobinuria may be present in acute Haemolytic anaemias.

Methaemalbuminaemia (Schumm's test) may be positive.

Haemosiderinuria, sometimes present.

Blood film: nucleated red cells present; increased reticulocytes, anspherocytosis and fragmentation of red cells.

Osmotic fragility—increased when spherocytes present.

Shortened red cell life span.

Acholuric jaundice (hereditary spherocytosis)

Age at which the disease is recognised ranged from infants to old age—but more usually in the younger age groups.

Haemoglobin normal, or mild anaemia, except in a crisis when it is very low.

P.C.V. reduced slightly if there is anaemia.

M.C.H.C. High (37–39 per cent).

Film: marked anisocytosis, with presence of very small darkly staining red cells (microspherocytes).

Reticulocytes increased.

Fragility of red cells in hypotonic saline is increased.

Serum bilirubin raised. (Indirect van den Bergh)

Urine Urobilinogen raised.

Haemoglobinopathies:

Thalassaemia major (homozygous state). Foetal haemoglobin (alkali resistant haemoglobin) positive, and forming 40–100% of total haemoglobin. Haemoglobin A_2 usually raised.

Thalassaemia minor (Heterozygous state). Haemoglobin F slightly raised (5-10% of total haemoglobin). Haemoglobin A_2 often raised.

Sickle cell trait (heterozygous state). Sickle cell slide test positive.

Sickle cell disease (homozygous state). Peripheral blood may show directly some sickle cells.

In these haemoglobinopathies the blood film shows target cells and haemoglobin electrophoresis separates haemoglobin A, A_2, F, S, D, E etc.

Leukaemias (chronic)

(Chronic myeloid and lymphatic leukaemia are the two of major importance. Other types are rarer.)

Haemoglobin low.

Leucocytes high (50,000 up to several hundred thousand).

Platelets vary according to the stage and type of disease.

E.S.R. raised.

Uric acid high.

Neutrophil alkaline phosphatase low in myeloid laukaemia.

Leukaemias (acute)

(Acute myeloblastic, lymphoblastic and monoblastic are the three commonest types).

Haemoglobin low.

Leucocytes raised (up to 100,000 often) or low (occasionally less than 1,000 in the subleukaemic variety).

Platelets low.

E.S.R. raised.

Uric acid high.

Marrow—'blast' cells predominate (these are the primitive cells of the bone marrow).

BLEEDING AND CLOTTING DISORDERS

Haemostasis is the preservation of an intact blood circulation. A defect of haemostasis will result in an abnormal tendency to bleed, and can be caused by faults in any of the following components:

1. Blood vessels.
2. Platelets.
3. Clotting factors.

Defects of these 3 components can cause haemorrhagic disorders as follows:

1. *Vascular defects* (capillary fragility)
(*a*) non-thrombocytopenic purpuras—e.g. scurvy, uraemia, macro-globulinaemia, drugs.
(*b*) Henoch Schonlein purpura.
(*c*) Senile purpura.
(*d*) hereditary haemorrhagic telangiectasia.

2. *Platelet defects*
(*a*) thrombocytopenia (primary).
(*b*) thrombocytopenia (secondary)—e.g. caused by drugs, leukaemia, aplastic anaemia, and bone marrow infiltration with malignant tissue as in secondary carcinomatosis, myelomatosis and the lymphoas.   m

3. *Coagulation defects*
   (*a*) haemophilia.
   (*b*) Christmas disease.
   (c) Fibrinogen deficiency and fibrinolysis. (e.g. obstetric causes where placental extracts in the circulation is responsible for precipitating the fibrinogen and therefore leading to deficiency of this protein for clotting purposes).
   (*d*) Liver disease.
   (*e*) Von Willebrand's disease.

Tests which may be requested
   Platelet count
   Prothrombin time
   Bleeding time
   Clotting time
   Partial Thromboplastin time
   Thromboplastin generation test
   Specific clotting factors.

MISCELLANEOUS.

Haemoglobinuria
   Spectroscopy reveals the characteristic bands of haemoglobin, If the urine is allowed to stand, there is conversion to *methaemoglobin* which has different spectroscopic characteristics.

Myoglobinuria.
Fresh urine is examined spectroscopically.

Hodgkins disease
Haemoglobin usually normal but may be low.
Direct Coombs test positive occasionally.
White cells variable in different stages.—Eosinophilia sometimes.
Platelets often decreased.

Methaemoglobinaemia, Sulphaemoglobinaemia, Carboxyhaemoglobinaemia
Spectroscopy of a dilution of haemolysed red cells reveals a weak characteristic absorption band in the red.

Polycythaemia Rubra vera
Red cells are raised (often 8/9 million/cmm.).
Haemoglobin is raised (18–24 G/100 ml).
M.C.H. often slightly reduced.
P.C.V. > 56%
M.C.V. lower normal range or slightly low.
Reticulocytes—upper normal, or slightly increased.
Red cells show slight anisocytosis and poikilocytosis, and often slight hypochromia.
White cells—12–20,000/cmm (slightly raised).
Leucocyte alkaline phosphatase increased.
Platelets raised 500,000—1,000,000/c.mm.
E.S.R. reduced.
Serum uric acid raised.
Bone marrow—hyperplasia.
Total blood volume is increased because of a red cell volume rise.

Secondary polycythaemia (to hypoxia)
Red cells increased.
White Cells and platelets normal.
Haemoglobin raised.
P.C.V. raised.
Reticulocytes slightly raised sometimes.
Red cells often microcytic.
Marrow—selective red cell hyperplasia.
Total blood volume raised because of a red cell volume rise.
Plasma volume normal or slightly reduced.

Cardiovascular system

Congestive cardiac failure
Plasma sodium and chloride fall, particularly if patient is on low salt diet. Plasma potassium falls with use of diuretics unless supplementary dietary potassium is given.

Tendency for blood urea to rise.

Proteinuria.

Serum albumin decreases and albumin/globulin ratio decreases.

Pyruvate metabolism test abnormal.

Essential hypertension
Slight rise of urinary catecholamines but this is much less than in the case of hypertension associated with phaeochromocytoma.

24 hour urinary vanillylmandelic acid (V.M.A.) (H.M.M.A.) excretion normal.

In the later stages of hypertension and in malignant hypertension there will be biochemical evidence of renal damage and failure. Differentiation must then be made from hypertension secondary to renal disease including unilateral renal disease.

Cardiac infarction
S.G.O.T. rises rapidly within a few hours and returns to normal within 2–3 days.

Serum lactic dehydrogenase rises and falls more slowly (normal in about 5 days). Specific isoenzyme pattern.

Transient rise in serum C.P.K. raised α–Hydroxybutyrate Dehydrogenase (H.B.D.)

Increase of serum globulins.

Moderate impairment of glucose tolerance for approximately 3 weeks.

Endocrine system

PITUITARY GLAND

Acromegaly and gigantism
Fasting blood sugar may be high. Impaired glucose tolerance with diabetes mellitus in some cases. No ketosis.

Increased insulin tolerance.

Raised serum inorganic phosphate.

Fasting serum growth hormone high with paradoxical rise during glucose tolerance test.

Hypopituitarism (including chromophobe adenoma)

Increased glucose tolerance with 'flattened curve'.

Marked increase of insulin sensitivity. Failure of the normal rise in Plasma growth hormone and cortisol to insulin induced hypoglycaemia.

Many biochemical features of hypothyroidism may be present including low B.M.R. and decreased thyroid radioactive iodine uptake, but serum cholesterol tends to remain normal. Thyroid function tests improve after course of thyrotrophin.

Many biochemical features of adrenocortical insufficiency may be present including low plasma cortisol, low urinary excretion of 17-oxosteroids, 17-oxogenic steriods and 17-hydroxycorticosteroids, but there is a rise after A.C.T.H. or Synacthen administration.

Metopirone test positive.

Failure to excrete water load normally is corrected after cortisone administration.

Pyrogen test positive.

Diminished excretion of urinary gonadotrophins.

Pituitary dwarfism

Failure to demonstrate a rise of plasma growth hormone following an adequate stimulus such as the administration of Bovril, (Ref 2.) or intravenous I.V. insulin sufficient to cause hypoglycaemia.

Diabetes insipidus (D I.)

Polyuria is very marked in the classical disease. If partial D.I. is present the urine volume will fall appreciably in later stages of dehydration.

Urine specific gravity and osmolality very low but may rise if dehydration becomes marked.

Plasma osmolality high.

Plasma sodium and chloride high.

Blood urea rises when dehydration is severe.

Administration of vasopressin tannate inhibits the diuresis in D.I. of pituitary origin but has no effect on nephrogenic D.I.

ADRENAL CORTEX

Cushing's syndrome (of adrenal origin)

Fasting blood sugar may be raised with glycosuria. Impaired glucose tolerance.

Increased insulin tolerance.

Raised plasma cortisol with failure of suppression after Dexamethasone and loss of diurnal rhythm.

Raised urine 17-oxosteroids, 17-oxogenic steroids and 17-hydroxycorticosteroids.

Decrease in plasma potassium with metabolic alkalosis in some cases.

Decrease in urine sodium excretion but increase in urine potassium excretion.

Plasma A.C.T.H. concentration is undetectable in Cushing's syndrome of adrenal origin.

In Cushing's disease in which there is a basophil adenoma of the pituitary gland plasma A.C.T.H. levels are high. Even higher levels are found in patients with ectopic production of A.C.T.H., e.g. carcinoma of the bronchus.

Adrenogenital syndrome in young adults

Increased excretion of urine total 17-hydroxycorticosteroids, oxosteroids and oxogenic steroids, which are suppressed to normal by replacement doses of cortisone.

Increased urine excretion of pregnanetriol which is also suppressed to normal by replacement doses of cortisone.

Primary hyperaldosteronism (Conn's syndrome)

Increased excretion of urinary aldosterone.

Raised serum sodium and lowered serum potassium. Metabolic alkalosis. Decreased urinary sodium excretion and increased potassium excretion. All these changes are reversed by administration of aldosterone antagonists.

Negative potassium balance.

Serum magnesium low.

Urine volume large.

Adrenocortical insufficiency

Low plasma cortisol.

Low urinary excretion of 17-oxosteroids, 17-oxogenic steroids and 17-hydroxycorticosteroids.

Low serum sodium and high serum potassium.

High urine sodium and low urine potassium.

Increased glucose tolerance.

A.C.T.H. stimulation test negative.

Failure to excrete water load normally is corrected after cortisone administration.

Blood urea rises slowly in late stages of the disease.

ADRENAL MEDULLA

Phaeochromocytoma

Fasting blood sugar may be high and associated with glycosuria.

Impaired glucose tolerance.

High urine excretion of catecholamines and vanillymandelic acid (V.M.A.) (H.M.M.A.) but these findings may be transient, and associated with exacerbations of hypertension.

Increased excretion in urine of 5-hydroxyindole acetic acid.

THYROID GLAND

Primary hyperthyroidism (thyrotoxicosis)

Raised B.M.R.

Low serum cholesterol.

Raised serum protein-bound-iodine.

Triiodothyronine resin uptake increased.

Raised thyroid radioactive iodine uptake, with failure of suppression with tri iodothyronine.

Decreased urinary radioactive iodine excretion.

Decreased glucose tolerance.

Primary hypothyroidism and myxoedema

Raised serum cholesterol.

Low protein bound iodine.

Low tri iodothyronine resin uptake.

Low thyroid radioactive iodine uptake with failure of stimulation with thyrotrophin (T.S.H.).

Increased urinary radioactive iodine excretion.

Cretinism due to primary thyroid deficiency

Low radioactive iodine uptake by thyroid gland with no increase after T.S.H. in most, but not all, forms of Cretinism.

Low Protein bound iodine.

Serum cholesterol very high.

Iodine deficiency goitre

Increased radioactive iodine uptake by thyroid gland which rapidly falls to normal after iodine is added to the diet.

Hashimoto's disease
Serum antibody tests to thyroid are positive.
Raised E.S.R.
Serum protein-bound iodine low.
B.M.R. low.
Serum cholesterol raised.
Thyroid radio active iodine uptake increased.
Serum globulins raised.

PARATHYROID GLANDS

Primary hyperparathyroidism
Fasting serum calcium may be slightly or markedly raised and is
not suppressed by cortisone administration.
High urinary calcium excretion.
Low fasting serum inorganic phosphate.
Raised serum alkaline phosphatase.
Urinary phosphate clearance increased.
Renal tubular reabsorption of phosphate decreased.
Phosphate excretion index increased.

Hypoparathyroidism
Fasting serum calcium low.
Urinary calcium excretion low or nil.
Fasting serum inorganic phosphate raised.
Urinary phosphate clearance decreased.
Renal tubular reabsorption of phosphate increased.
Phosphate excretion index decreased.
With the Ellsworth-Howard test there is a phosphate diuresis
which differentiates hypoparathyroidism from pseudohypopara-
thyroidism.See Chapter 3 p.50

Pseudohypoparathyroidism
Biochemical features of hypoparathyroidism but Ellsworth-Howard
test (p. 50) shows failure of reponse to parathormone.

MISCELLANEOUS

Tumours of the ovary
Arrhenoblastoma. Increased urinary excretion of 17-oxosteroids
not suppressed by dexamethasone.
Granulosa cell tumour. Increased urinary excretion of oestrogens.

Kidneys and excretory system

Acute and chronic renal failure (uraemia)

Blood urea raised.
Plasma potassium raised.
Serum creatinine raised.
Blood pH falls and alkali reserve falls. (Metabolic acidosis.)
Serum phosphate raised.
Plasma osmolality raised.
Glomerular filtration rate and creatinine clearance lowered.
Urine findings depend on the cause of the renal failure.

Acute nephritis (type I)

Blood findings as in renal failure.
Urine contains blood and protein.
Urine volume low.
Urine specific gravity may be high due to protein content but urine urea and osmolality low.

Acute tubular necrosis

Blood findings as in renal failure.
In early stages urine volume low. Proteinuria. Low urine urea.
Specific gravity 1·010 (osmolality approximately 300 ± 100 mosmols/kg).
In later stages urine volume rises but urea content remains low even in presence of high blood urea. Plasma potassium may fall rapidly during this stage.

Chronic nephritis

Blood findings as in renal failure but in addition serum albumin decreases and globulin fractions increase.
Urine volume large with impairment of concentration and dilution leading eventually to fixity of specific gravity at 1·010 (osmolality 300 ± 100mosmols/kg).
Proteinuria.
Urine urea low even in presence of high blood urea.

Nephrotic syndrome (nephrosis) (type II nephaitis)

In the later stages many of the blood findings of renal failure are present. In addition:
Raised serum cholesterol and raised total lipid.

Decreased serum total protein and albumin but rise oFα_2 and β globulins.

Thymol and Kunkel turbidity raised.

Urine protein concentration very high with specific gravity disproportionately higher than osmolality.

De Toni-Fanconi syndrome

Biochemically this syndrome combines the features of renal glycosuria, phosphaturic rickets, renal tubular acidosis together with amino-aciduria, and increased potassium loss by the kidney.

Cystinosis

Cystine crystals detectable in tissues particularly bone marrow.

Many features of the De Toni-Fanconi syndrome (vide supra) may be present.

Orthostatic proteinuria

Protein occurs in the urine regularly after standing and is not present in the early morning urine specimen.

Carcinoma of prostate

Raised serum formol stable acid phosphatase.

Increased serum alkaline phosphatase indicates presence of secondary deposits in bone or liver.

Renal Tubular acidosis

Urine pH usually greater than 6·5. Does not fall below 5·6 after administration of ammonium chloride.

Low urine titratable acid. Failure of urine concentration.

Biochemical changes in plasma are those of metabolic acidosis, i.e. reduced plasma alkali reserve, and increased plasma chloride.

Decreased plasma phosphate and increased urine phosphate excretion (with appropriate changes in tubular phosphate indices (p. 49) and raised plasma alkaline phosphatase. p. 49.

Renal glycosuria

Glucose appears in urine at blood levels below 180 mg/100 ml which is the normal reival threshold for glucose.

Metabolic diseases.

galactosaemia

Increased level of reducing substances in blood (galactose) but low blood glucose in untreated cases.

Proteinuria and increased reducing substances in urine (galactose).

Paper chromatography of urine shows presence of galactose.
Amino-aciduria.
The red cell galactose-1-phosphate uridyl transferase activity is reduced.

Metabolic acidosis
    Blood pH ↓
    Urine pH ↓ except in renal tubular defect.
    Alkali reserve ↓ $PaCO_2$ ↓
    Standard bicarbonate ↓
    Plasma chloride ↑
    Buffer base ↓
    Base excess ↓

Metabolic alkalosis
    Blood pH ↑ $PaCO_2$ ↑
    Urine pH ↑
    Alkali reserve ↑
    Standard bicarbonate ↑
    Plasma chloride ↓
    Buffer base ↑
    Base excess ↑

Respiratory acidosis
    Blood pH ↓ $PaCO_2$ ↑
    Urine pH ↓
    Alkali reserve ↑
    Standard bicarbonate ↑
    Plasma chloride ↓
    Buffer base ↑
    Base excess ↑

Respiratory alkalosis
    Blood pH ↑
    Urine pH ↑ $PaCO_2$ ↓
    Alkali reserve ↓
    Standard bicarbonate ↓
    Plasma chloride ↑
    Buffer base ↓
    Base excess ↓

Miscellaneous disorders

Sarcoidosis
Serum calcium sometimes raised but falls to normal after cortisone administration. Serum alkaline phosphatase sometimes raised.

Plasma proteins increased, particularly globulin fraction with decrease in albumin/globulin ratio and increased thymol and Kunkel turbidity.
Urine calcium excretion sometimes increased.

Macroglobulinaemia (Waldenström's disease)
Sia test positive.
Increased total serum protein, and increased serum viscosity.
On electrophoresis there is a band which remains stationary at the point of application.
Serum macroglobulin content increased (ultracentrifugation.)
Immunoglobulin M. Raised. (Immuno electrophoresis.)

Myelomatosis
Serum total protein raised or Globulin fraction increased with decrease in albumin/globulin ratio. A discrete band in globulin fraction on electrophoresis.
Abnormal thymol turbidity and Kunkel tests.
Serum calcium increased.
Serum alkaline phosphatase increased.
Increased urinary calcium.

Cryoglobulinaemia
Increase in serum globulin fraction.
The blood is taken in a warm syringe. The cryoglobulin will precipitate out as a white opalescence on allowing the separated serum to stand and cool.

Lead intoxication
Whole blood lead greater than 80 μgm/100 ml.
Urinary lead excretion on several 24 hour specimens greater than 80 μgm/24 hours.
A raised blood lead and increased urine excretion of lead may be present in subjects who have been exposed to lead but who have not developed clinical features of intoxication.
Urinary lead excretion increases markedly after E.D.T.A. treatment.
Urine coproporphyrin III and uroporphyrin III increased.
Urine amino-acid excretion increased.

Carcinoidosis

Urine excretion of 5-hydroxyindole acetic acid (5H.I.A.A.) markedly increased.

Urinary excretion of 4-hydroxy-3-methoxy mandelic acid (V.M.A.) (H.M.M.A.) increased in some cases.

The patient's diet must have contained no bananas for several days prior to this assay being carried out.

Haemochromatosis

Serum iron raised.

Serum iron combining capacity saturated.

Fasting blood sugar may be raised and glycosuria may be present.

Decreased glucose tolerance.

Urinary excretion of 17-oxosteroids decreased.

Alkaptonuria

Urine darkens on standing.

Tests for reducing compounds (e.g. Benedict's test) positive but no glucose present in urine by glucose oxidase test.

No other sugars present in urine on paper chromatography.

Homogentisic acid present in urine.

PORPHYRIAS

Acute intermittent porphyria

Increased excretion of urinary porphobilinogen, uroporphyrin and coproporphyrin, during attacks.

Increased urinary excretion of δ-amino-laevulinic acid even between attacks.

Faecal porphyrins present particularly during attacks.

Plasma non-fluorescent.

Porphyria cutanea tarda

Increased excretion of urinary porphobilinogen, uroporphyrin and coproporphyrin during attacks.

Faecal porphyrins present between attacks.

Plasma fluorescent.

Congenital erythropoietic porphyria

Urine porphobilinogen not increased.

Increased excretion of urinary uroporphyrin and coproporphyrin.

Faecal porphyrins increased.

Plasma fluorescent.

Kwashiorkor
Reduced serum total protein and decreased albumin/globulin ratio.
Reduced blood sugar, urea and serum α-amino nitrogen, copper and caeruloplasmin.
Amino-aciduria.

Vitamin B₁ deficiency and Wernicke's encephalopathy
Pyruvate metabolism test abnormal.
Red cell transketolase activity reduced, with an increase following the addition of thiamine pyrophosphate.

Scurvy
Reduced plasma and white cell vitamin C content.
Vitamin C saturation test positive.

Vitamin D intoxication
Raised serum calcium which returns to normal after cortisone administration.
Increased urinary excretion of calcium.
Serum alkaline phosphatase and inorganic phosphate normal.

Metabolic response to trauma (including surgical operations)
Serum G.O.T., L.D.H. and C.P.K. all rise temporarily as a result of tissue injury.
Plasma fibrinogen rises.
Blood urea often rises slightly, Rise of blood sugar.
There is sodium and water retention, with a fall in urine volume even in the presence of liberal fluid intake. Urinary potassium excretion rises.
The body is in negative nitrogen balance.
Rise in plasma cortisol with increased urinary excretion of steriods and 17-hydroxycorticosteroids.
Slight proteinuria and ketonuria sometimes present.

Collagen diseases
Raised total protein in blood with decrease of A/G ratio.
Raised E.S.R.
L. E. Latex test positive.
Haemolytic anaemia.
Leucopenia.
L.E. cell test positive.
Rose Waaler test positive.
Serum antinuclear factor positive.

PREGNANCY

Some biochemical changes of importance in normal pregnancy
Mild anaemias.
Fall in serum iron.
Fall in A/G ratio.
Mild proteinuria.
Reducing substances in urine: glucose and lactose.
Decreased glucose tolerance.
Raised urinary gonadotrophins (chorionic).
Raised urine pregnanediol
Raised urine 17-oxosteroids and oxgenic steroids.
Raised blood volume.
Raised P.B.I.
Raised B.M.R.
Raised serum cholesterol.
Raised plasma fibrinogen.
Raised E.S.R.
Raised total W.C.C.

Nervous system (see also cerebrospinal fluid, p. 42)

Subarachnoid haemorrhage
Glucose tolerance impaired for about 3 weeks. Sometimes fasting blood sugar is raised with glycosuria. Blood in CSF with xanthochromia.

Subacute combined degeneration of spinal cord (and pernicious anaemia)
Serum vitamin B_{12} low ($<$180 $\mu\mu$gm/ml).
Schilling test (Part 1) shows very poor absorption of radioactive vitamin B_{12} but normal absorption following addition of Intrinsic Factor. (Part 2).
Abnormal pyruvate metabolism test.

Friedreich's ataxia
10 per cent patients show decreased glucose tolerance.

A-β lipoproteinaemia
Very low serum cholesterol ($<$ 100 mg/100 ml.)
Decrease in low density lipoproteins.
Very low fasting serum triglycerides.
Abnormal pattern on lipoprotein electrophoresis with absent β band.
Biochemical features of idiopathic steatorrhoea.
Acanthrocytes in peripheral blood.

Peripheral neuropathy
Associated with diabetes mellitus, subacute combined degeneration of spinal cord, idiopathic steatorrhoea, collagen diseases, vitamin B_1 deficiency.
See appropriate headings.

Myasthenia gravis
Low plasma pseudocholinesterase activity.

Guillain-Barré syndrome
C.S.F. Protein markedly raised. Normal cell count.

Multiple sclerosis
C.S.F. Cell count normal or slightly raised lymphocyte count.
C.S.F. total protein usually normal or slightly raised. Globulin disproportionately raised giving positive Pandy test.
Lange—Paretic curve may be present.

Meningitis
Purulent.
C.S.F. protein raised. Raised white cell count (mainly poly-morphonuclear leucocytes.)
Bacterial organisms present in smear and in culture.
Low C.S.F. sugar.
Blood Polymorphonuclear leucocytosis. Blood culture may be positive.

Lymphocytic:	C.S.F. raised lymphocyte count.
	C.S.F. normal sugar.
	C.S.F. slightly raised protein.
Tuberculous:	C.S.F. raised lymphocyte count.
	C.S.F. raised protein.
	C.S.F. low sugar (in late stages).
	C.S.F. tubercle bacilli may be found on smear: may be cultured on media or in guinea-pig.

Wilson's disease
Serum caeruloplasmin reduced.
Serum copper reduced.
Urine copper excretion increased.
Amino-aciduria.
Low serum uric acid.

Abnormal pyruvate metabolism test which fails to revert to normal with vitamin B_1 therapy.

Refsum's disease
Phytanic acid present in abnormal amounts in serum, and C.S.F.

Acute polymyositis
Serum C.P.K. raised.
Serum G.O.T. raised.
Blood E.S.R. raised.

McArdle's disease and other glycogen storage diseases of muscle
Ischaemic exercise lactate test positive.
Myoglobin may be present in urine after exercise.

Metachromatic leucodystrophy.
Increased sulphatide excretion in urine.
Intracellular metachromatic material present in centrifuged urine deposits.

MUSCULAR DYSTROPHIES

Duchenne muscular dystrophy (X-linked recessive)
The most useful enzyme to assay is C.P.K. This is markedly raised particularly in the earlier stages of the severe form of the disease.
Raised in the slowly progressive benign (Becker) type.
Raised serum and urine creatine.

Progressive muscular dystrophy autosomal recessive
High serum C.P.K. levels in patients but not in carriers.

Limb-girdle muscular dystrophy
Serum enzymes frequently moderately raised in patients but not in carriers.
(Note that in neurogenic muscular atrophy enzymes are usually normal.)

Dystrophia myotonica
Serum enzymes slightly raised in 50 per cent cases.

PERIODIC PARALYSIS

Hypokalaemic type
Serum potassium low during attacks.
Low serum potassium may be induced by high carbohydrate and high sodium chloride intake particularly if combined with insulin administration.
Attacks associated with low serum potassium are prevented by low sodium chloride intake in the diet.

Hyperkalaemic (Adynamia episodica hereditaria)
Serum potassium high during attacks.

Respiratory system

Pulmonary infarction
Rise of serum G.O.T., aldolase and L.D.H. (with specific L.D.H. isoenzyme pattern).
Increase of urine urobilinogen.

Pleural effusion
Transudates have a low protein content <1·5 G/100 ml.
Exudates have a high protein content > 2.0 G/100 ml and may contain fibrin clot.

Skeletal system (*see also parathyroid glands*)
Paget's disease of bone (osteitis deformans)
Serum calcium and inorganic phosphate normal.
Alkaline phosphatase high or very high with characteristic pattern on isoenzyme electrophoresis.
Increased urinary calcium excretion may be present.

Osteomalacia and rickets of dietary origin
Low serum calcium and inorganic phosphate.
Raised serum alkaline phosphatase.
Low urine calcium excretion.
Increased faecal calcium excretion.

osteomalacia and rickets due to renal tubular defect and vitamin D resistant rickets

Serum calcium normal or low.
Serum inorganic phosphate low.
Serum alkaline phosphatase raised.

Urinary calcium low.
Urinary inorganic phosphate high.
Faecal calcium output increased.
Glycosuria and increased urine amino-acid excretion may occur.

Osteoporosis

Serum calcium, inorganic phosphate and alkaline phosphatase normal.

Urinary calcium excretion may be raised.

Secondary carcinomatosis of bone

Serum calcium may be raised.

Serum alkaline phosphatase raised with characteristic pattern on isoenzyme electrophoresis.

Serum 5-nucleotidase normal.

Urinary excretion of calcium raised.

Gout

Serum uric acid raised.

APPENDIX A

Preparation of patients for special tests where no specific instructions are given by the laboratory

If specific instructions are not issued by the laboratory it may be assumed that no special preparation of the patient is required nor special precautions needed in the collection of samples. In general, however, the following points should receive attention.

a. Collect at least 5–6 ml blood in adults, using minimal venous stasis, i.e. with the tourniquet on for only a few seconds in order to identify the vein and then released as soon as blood commences to enter the syringe. The patient must always be carefully observed for signs of fainting.

b. Avoid the use of very fine needles and draw the blood slowly. Remove needle before transferring blood into the appropriate dry container. These precautions help to minimize haemolysis.

c. If the bottle contains an anticoagulant mix gently by inverting immediately two or three times. *Do not shake.*

d. Keep away from radiators and despatch as soon as possible to the laboratory.

Patient fasting. Water only is allowed or even encouraged from 10 p.m. the previous evening until the test is completed and all samples have been collected. Usually the patient is kept at rest in bed, and smoking is best avoided.

Nil by mouth. As for 'fasting' but water is not allowed either. Orally administered drugs are sometimes omitted but clearly there will be exceptions to this in which case specific instructions should be obtained.

Patient under basal conditions. As for 'nil by mouth' but in addition, after being allowed up for five minutes only to toilet (not for washing or shaving) at say 6.30–7 a.m. the patient returns to lie at *absolute rest* in bed for 2–3 hours until the test is completed. No smoking is allowed.

These conditions are required for pyruvate and lactate determinations and the blood samples will be collected by the laboratory staff and pipetted at the bedside.

For Basal Metabolic rate (B.M.R.) the patient must be at *Total* rest and in a separate room.

Collection of specimens

Blood samples for which special precautions are required

Alkali reserve and total CO_2 content of blood. After blood is withdrawn, the sample is gently injected via a second widebore needle below the surface of liquid paraffin previously placed in a heparin tube. The tube is kept vertical and is not inverted.

Ammonia. Blood for ammonia concentration will be collected by the laboratory staff. Generally the patient should not be fasting and frequently should have been on a high protein diet for about three days (note that this may be dangerous in patients with impaired liver function).

Calcium. Particular care is required to minimize venous stasis. Transient (a few seconds) use of the lightly applied tourniquet to identify the vein is permitted. The tourniquet is removed immediately after puncturing the vein and blood has started to enter the syringe. Blood is placed in a clean acid-washed tube.

Cortisol (11-hydroxycorticosteroids). The exact time of collection must be noted (may be midnight or 8 a.m.). Ideally blood should be taken into a special heparin tube (not inverted) and plasma separated within an hour and pipetted into containers placed in laboratory 'deep freeze' at $-20°C$.

Creatine phosphokinase C.P.K. Attention should be paid as to whether the patient has recently taken exercise.

Insulin and Growth Hormone. Blood is collected into heparin tubes and the cells separated at once by centrifugation in the laboratory. The plasma is kept in the 'deep freeze' at−20°C. If transport to another laboratory is required, the plasma must be sent in a thermos flask containing ice.

Iron. Blood will be collected by laboratory staff with special syringes into special containers.

Lactate, pyruvate. The patient must be basal. Minimum venous stasis. Blood is pipetted by laboratory staff at the bedside.

Lead, mercury and copper. Special syringes and containers are required from the laboratory.

Phosphate. Blood is collected into a heparin tube and despatched at once to the laboratory for immediate separation of plasma from cells.

Potassium. Plasma potassium values are invalidated if there is visible evidence of haemolysis.

Protein bound iodine. Do not use iodine containing compounds to clean the skin. During collection of blood and separation of cells, care must be taken to avoid contamination with *traces* of iodine. The patient should preferably be on a fish free diet for three days before blood is taken and care taken to ensure that the patient has no medications which contain iodine. Contrast media used in Radiology may interfere with this test.

Sugar. Collect into a fluoride bottle.

Urine samples

24 hour urine collections. These often commence in the early morning (say 8 a.m.) but may in fact start at any time. The bladder is emptied (either with patient standing or sitting or if in bed with suprapubic pressure) at the time stated and the urine *discarded*. All specimens are then collected as they are passed up to and including the same time next day, the final specimen (8 a.m. in the example) being placed into the container.

Note that the collection bottle often contains preservative.

Early morning specimens. For biochemical tests usually only part of the first specimen passed in the morning is required. This need not be a midstream specimen and need be collected only into a clean dry (non-sterile) universal container. If vaginal discharge is present a catheter specimen of urine may be required.

Casual specimens. As for early morning specimens but may be collected at any time.

INSTRUCTIONS FOR URINE COLLECTION IN SOME SPECIAL TESTS

(Most other tests require casual, early morning or 24 hour collections without preservative.)

δ-*amino-laevulinic acid.* 24 hour urine collection. Bottle contains dilute acetic acid.

Calcium excretion. 24 hour urine collection. Bottle contains dilute hydrochloric acid.

Catecholamines. 24 hour urine collection, into a dark bottle containing dilute sulphuric acid.

Gonadotrophins. 24 hour urine collection. Bottle contains methiolate.

5-hydroxyindole acetic acid. 24 hour urine collection into a dark bottle containing glacial acetic acid. Patients must have been on banana free diet for 3–4 days.

Lead, copper and mercury. 24 hour urine collection in specially provided plastic container. The lid must be only removed momentarily and not placed anywhere except directly back on the container. This is to avoid possible contamination. Urine must be passed directly into the container with the use of the specially provided plastic funnel.

PORPHOBILINOGEN AND PORPHYRINS

Porphobilinogen. (*a*). Casual specimen sent to the laboratory *at once*.

(*b*). 24 hour urine collection into a dark bottle containing solid sodium carbonate.

Porphyrins (*uroporphyrin and coproporphyrin*). Either (*a*) Casual specimen or (*b*) 24 hour urine collection.

Tryptophan load test (Xanthurenic acid). 24 hour urine collection preserved with 25 ml normal hydrochloric acid.

Urea, creatine, creatinine. 24 hour urine collection. Bottle contains crystals of thymol or a few ml of toluene.

*Vanillylmandilic acid (V.M.A.)*H.M.M.A. 24 hour urine collection. Bottle contains fairly strong hydrochloric acid.

Vitamin C (for saturation test). All urine passed between 4 and 6 hours after oral vitamin C administration is collected into a dark bottle containing 20 ml glacial acetic acid and sent *at once* for analysis.

Stool samples

Faecal fat analysis. All samples collected in cellophane and placed in plastic cartons for, at the very least, 4 and preferably 6 days. If markers are used at the beginning and end of the test, both should be passed completely.

Aperients should be avoided during the test, and ideally a diet of approximately known fat content should be given. If a fat balance study is being made, the exact fat content of the diet must be known.

Faecal porphyrins. Part of any stool should be sent to the laboratory. The patient should have been on a chlorophyll-free diet (no green vegetables or lettuce) for 4–5 days.

Occult blood in stools. Patient should have been on a diet free of red meat 3 days before the test.

The cerebrospinal fluid

Cerebrospinal fluid should be collected into two clean, dry sterile containers and sent at once to the laboratory. A total volume of *at least* 6 ml should be provided. In addition collection into a fluoride bottle should be made if sugar estimation is required.

Other specimens

Gastric aspirate for test meals see p. 51.

Collection of samples from patients suspected of having been poisoned (including acute alcoholic coma)

Specimens should be obtained as early as possible, preferably just prior to administration of antidote.

About 20 ml blood collected into a tightly stoppered Heparin tube is satisfactory for most tests including blood alcohol. If sugar assays are required an additional sample should be collected into a fluoride bottle.

Urine (at least 50 ml) should be collected into a clean, dry universal container.

Stomach aspirate. The whole of the stomach aspirate taken before washing out the stomach must be kept. It should be uncontaminated by antidote.

Principles of Tolerance Tests and Clearance Tests

For details of particular tests see Chapter 3 "Function tests."
During tolerance tests in which patients are given a 'biochemical stimulus', e.g. a standard oral glucose load or an intravenous insulin injection points in the management of patients and in the collection of specimens require special attention though the details will vary with the particular test.

The following general points should be noted:

1. Frequently patients require special preparation, e.g. fasting, no smoking and may have to be placed on a special diet for 2–3 days prior to the test.

2. These investigations vary in length from, say, 20 minutes up to several hours, during which the patient stays in bed and apart from the test itself remains otherwise basal. There are, however, a few exceptions to this general rule.

3. It is extremely important that patients should be particularly closely observed during these tests as they sometimes become temporarily unwell as a result of the test which may have to be rapidly terminated (e.g. administration of intravenous glucose to patients rendered unduly hypoglycaemic during an Insulin Tolerance Test or a Tolbutamide Tolerance Test.) Thus the specific remedy for each test should be immediately available.

4. The accuracy of specimen collection during tolerance and clearance tests is particularly important and the timing may be critical to within one minute. Urine collections of small volume are often made over short periods of time and any inaccuracies will therefore be even more serious than usual. The bladder must be completely emptied after each collection. Tolerance tests are often un-

pleasant for the patient and it is important that they should not have to be repeated.

5. A clearance test is one in which a theoretical figure is calculated for the volume of blood passing through the kidney in unit time (usually 1 minute) which is completely cleared of some substance. Thus a urine collection over a specified time (often of the order of 1–2 hours but occasionally 24 hours) is made and blood is taken at the mid-point in time. All the statements about collection of specimens for tolerance tests apply to clearance tests. Sometimes the substance, the clearance of which is being measured, is administered to the patient at the beginning of the test.

Ward Sideroom Testing

For biochemical purposes ward sideroom testing should be confined to examination of the urine. Much valuable information may be obtained by quick and accurate testing of the urine on the ward particularly with emergency hospital admissions. Day to day testing is also important with other patients, especially in the case of diabetics and patients with kidney disease.

Much time can be saved too, in out-patient and casualty departments, antenatal clinics and in general practice by 'on-the-spot' urine testing.

The 'classical' methods of urine testing have tended to be replaced by commercial 'kits' which are satisfactory for many purposes if there is strict adherence to the manufacturer's instructions. Nevertheless, the older methods sometimes give more information and should be used where indicated.

Practical details of urine testing (*for further details see Ref* 3).

Appearance.

Pale yellow	Normal
Dark yellow or brown	Concentrated urine. Many drugs. Bile pigments. Methaemalbumin Melanin.
'Port wine colour' or red	Porphyrins. Phenolphthalein.
Bluish Green	Methylene blue. Diagnex blue.
Black	Melanin. Cresol poisoning.
Darkens on standing	Porphobilinogen. Homogentisic acid (rapidly darkens when made alkaline) Melanin.
Reddish and cloudy (smoky)	Blood.
Dark Orange	Phenindione Therapy.

Red precipitate	Urates (dissolve with heat or acid).
White precipitate	Phosphates (dissolve with acid).
Gelatinous deposit	Mucus.

Smell.

See inborn errors of metabolism. Appendix H. p. 105.

Specific gravity.

This is measured with a urinometer at 15°C, making sure that the instrument is absolutely freely suspended and that there are no air bubbles in the urine. The reading must be taken looking horizontally at the bottom of the meniscus.

N.R. 1·002–1·032.

pH.

Test with indicator paper.

N.R. 4·5–7·8.

Protein

(*a*). *Boiling test.* Fill a test tube two-thirds full of urine. Test with litmus paper and if alkaline add 10 per cent acetic acid drop by drop with mixing until just acid (litmus paper turning from blue to red). If already acid render just alkaline with dilute sodium hydroxide and adjust again with dilute acetic acid.

Incline the tube at an angle and heat the upper portion examining against a dark background for any precipitate which indicates the presence of protein or phosphates. The latter will disappear after the addition of more acid and further boiling. A persistent cloud indicates the presence of protein (approximately 20 mg/100 ml). A heavy precipitate of protein should be allowed to settle for 30 minutes. As a very rough guide, if at the end of this time the precipitate occupies half the test tube the urine contains protein of the order of 1 gram/100 ml, and if one-eighth of the tube a concentration of the order of 200 mg/100 ml.

A faint cloud of protein which redissolves on boiling and precipitates again on cooling (the urine may be filtered while hot) indicates the presence of Bence-Jones protein.

(b). *Sulphosalicylic acid test*. Add a few drops of 20 per cent sulphosalicylic acid to about 5 ml of filtered urine. A white precipitate indicates the presence of protein. Occasionally a false positive result will be obtained in patients who have recently been given radio-opaque preparations for radiological examinations: Some drugs will also produce a false positive.

(c). *Albustix*. Test according to manufacturer's instructions.

Quantitative assay of urine protein should be carried out by the laboratory on a 24 hour urine specimen.

There are very many causes of proteinuria including many types of acute and chronic disease of the kidney and its blood vessels, urinary tract infection, congestive heart failure and severe hypertension.

Any condition causing blood to be present in the urine will give rise to a positive test for protein. In women a catheter specimen of urine may be necessary to exclude traces of vaginal discharge.

During pregnancy the urine frequently contains a small amount of protein but if this increases it may be indicative of disease.

In young adults orthostatic proteinuria which disappears from urine collected after lying down is of no significance.

Bence-Jones protein is present in the urine of patients with myelomatosis and chronic myeloid leukaemia.

Blood

Haemastix. Test according to manufacturer's instructions.

Positive reaction indicates the presence of whole blood or haemoglobin. There are very many causes of blood in the urine and it is essential to remember that this is always an important and significant finding.

Glucose and reducing substances

Benedict's test. Eight drops of urine are added to 5 ml of Benedict's reagent, the mixture boiled for 2 minutes and allowed to cool. A precipitate indicates the presence of a reducing substance. If this is glucose, a very rough guide to its concentration may be obtained from the colour of the precipitate.

Light green turbidity   100–500 mg/100 ml.

Darker green precipitate	500 mg–1 G/100 ml.
Yellow precipitate	1·0–2·0 G/100 ml.
Reddish orange precipitate	greater than 2·0 G/100 ml.

Many reducing substances other than glucose can give a positive test (see Clinitest, Appendix H. p.105).

If a reducing substance is present but at the same time the supernatant turns black during the test, this indicates the presence of excess homogentisic acid and a diagnosis of alkaptonuria.

Clinitest. Test according to manufacturer's instructions.

Clinistix. Test according to manufacturer's instructions. This test is specific for glucose in urine. Occasionally a urine will give a positive result with Clinistix and a negative result with Clinitest. This is on account of the greater sensitivity of the Clinistix and indicates the presence of glucose in concentrations of less than 250 mg/100 ml. Excess vitamin C in urine may give false negative.

Ketones

Acetest. Test according to manufacturer's instructions.

Ferric chloride test. See section 'Inborn errors of metabolism'.

The conditions most commonly giving rise to ketones in the urine are diabetic ketosis and prolonged starvation or vomiting.

Bilirubin

Ictotest. Test according to manufacturer's instructions. Positive in acute hepatitis and obstructive jaundice.

Urobilinogen and porphobilinogen

To 1 ml of fresh urine add 1 ml Ehrlich's reagent and mix. After 2 minutes add 2 ml saturated sodium acetate solution and again mix. Then add 2 ml of a 3 : 1 mixture of Amyl alcohol/Benzyl alcohol. Shake well and allow the layers to separate. A brown colour in the upper layer indicates the presence of urobilinogen and a pink colour in the lower layer suggests the presence of porphobilinogen. If any colour does remain in the lower layer extraction with the alcohol mixture should be repeated and only if a pink colour persists is the presence of porphobilinogen confirmed.

Excess urobilinogen is presenti n the urine in haemolytic anaemias and the early phases of jaundice due to infective hepatitis. It is absent in cases of complete biliary obstruction.

The presence of any detectable porphobilinogen points to a diagnosis of porphyria and is particularly useful in the diagnosis of attacks of acute intermittent porphyria.

Notes on Intravenous Infusions

Intravenous infusions of blood, plasma or plasma substitutes, electrolytes and fat emulsions provide an extremely effective method of preventing and treating biochemical disorders in patients who are unable to take food or fluids by mouth. Occasionally infusions are also used for purely diagnostic purposes. A patient's clinical state can change dramatically for better or worse in a matter of an hour or so as a result of intravenous fluid therapy. Only rarely is fluid administered subcutaneously (with the help of hyalase) or per rectum. In unconcious patients, provided there is no disorder of the gastro-intestinal tract, fluid is best administered by gastric tube (see Appendix F, p. 100).

The brief notes that follow are intended as a practical guide to those left in charge of an intravenous infusion.

1. An intravenous infusion (I.V.F.) either by percutaneous needle or 'cut down' on a vein should run continuously; it should never be turned off except momentarily when changing bottles, and if it stops the medical officer in charge should be called at once. The rate should be carefully controlled and under no circumstances should fluid ever be 'blown' in under pressure.

2. Calculations should be based on the metric system using infusion bottles of 500 ml (0·5 litre) or 1,000 ml (1·0 litre) and clear instructions should be available at all times concerning the 'fluid regime' for the next few hours. Thus instructions must be left as to what the next bottle is to be, when it is to be through by, and whether it is to contain any additional factors such as extra potassium, vitamins, or antibiotics. The bottle must never be allowed to 'run dry'.

3. Fluid balance charts are particularly crucial during I.V.F. It

must be quite clear as to whether the fluid from a given bottle is entered on the chart when the bottle is started or when it has finished. The preferred system is to enter it when the bottle has finished. Urine volumes must be accurately measured and charted at once, as must any vomitus, liquid stools or gastric aspirations.

4. Fluids available. Apart from blood and packed cells, fluids available for I.V.F. may be classified as follows:

(a). 'Plasma expanders'—Plasma, dextran. These remain within the vascular compartment contributing to the blood volume and helping to maintain the blood pressure. Reconstituted dried plasma is frequently used but carries the risk of transmitting infective hepatitis. Dextrans are polyglucoses obtained by the fermentation of sucrose. They sometimes create difficulties when it becomes necessary to cross match blood for a patient who has received them. Thus blood for cross matching should be taken before dextran is administered.

(b). Solutions of electrolytes. These include normal saline, $\frac{1}{5}$ normal saline in dextrose, Darrow's solution for acidosis, Darrow's solution for alkalosis, Hartmann's solution, hypertonic saline and isotonic ($\frac{1}{6}$ molar) sodium lactate. Many other preparations are available for replacement of gastric or intestinal fluids. The basic principles underlying all these electrolyte preparations, however, are (1) the replacement of lost water, (2) correction of lost (or the anticipated loss of) sodium and potassium, (3) the correction of acid-base disorders.

(c). 5 per cent dextrose. This is used when it is necessary to administer water to patients who are suffering from dehydration. Water itself or solutions hypotonic compared with plasma cannot be given intravenously, as they will cause haemolysis of blood cells. Isotonic solutions such as 5 per cent dextrose in water or hypertonic solutions do not cause this effect. The dextrose content is insufficient to contribute materially to the patient's calorie requirements.

(d). Fat emulsions. These are a useful method of supplying calories, one litre of 20 per cent Intralipid for example supplying 2,000 calories. These solutions must be given slowly and must not be allowed to become mixed with other infusions. Blood for biochemical tests should be taken before the day's fat infusion is started, as the extreme lipaemia produced interferes with some tests.

5. 'Additives'. Factors sometimes added to I.V.F. include certain antibiotics, water soluble vitamins and extra potassium salts, as prescribed. These may only be added to 5 per cent dextrose infusions

and to *some* electrolyte infusions (vide infra) and **never** to blood, plasma, dextran or fat emulsions. Incompatibilities must also be avoided with double infusions. Full aseptic precautions are necessary when adding to infusions.

Particular care is necessary in the case of potassium salts. No intravenous infusion should contain a higher concentration of potassium than 40 mEq/L as higher concentrations than this may cause cardiac arrest. Moreover, the rate of infusion of potassium-containing-solutions must be carefully controlled, and must be stopped in the event of the patient developing urinary suppression. It must be remembered that Darrow's solution already contains the maximum concentration of potassium and *no further addition of potassium salts to this solution can be made.*

(Note 1·0 G potassium chloride = 13·5 mEq potassium. Hence 1·5 G potassium chloride (7·5 ml of 20 per cent solution) is the *maximum* amount which can be added to 500 ml of intravenous infusion or 3 G (15 ml of 20 per cent solution) to 1 litre.)

6. Blood samples for analysis should not be taken from the veins of a limb in which an intravenous infusion has been set up.

APPENDIX F

Notes on Tube Feeding

A normal, average daily diet for an adult man consists of approximately 2,500–3,000 calories and 70 G protein. Very wide variations occur however, manual workers requiring higher calorie and protein intakes than sedentary workers, and men more than women.

Patients not infrequently require tube feeding while in hospital. This may be on account of the post-operative state, prolonged unconsciousness, or for psychiatric reasons. It is important that these patients should receive adequate nutrition together with vitamin supplements.

Attention must be paid to the volume of the feed, the protein, carbohydrate, fat, mineral and vitamin contents. It is also desirable that tube feeds should be palatable in view of the possibility of some regurgitation occurring and the desirability of changing over to oral feeding as soon as possible.

In the past one of the commonest errors in tube feeding has been the administration of too much protein particularly when using proprietary preparations. In some instances (for example cases of burns) a high protein intake is necessary but in many patients a high protein intake will not lead to a positive nitrogen balance and the increased osmotic load will result in an osmotic diuresis, dehydration (sometimes with hypernatremia) and a mounting blood urea. This is seen particularly in unconscious patients who are unable to complain of thirst. Moreover it must not be assumed that patients are able to achieve maximal urinary concentration.

As a general guide, a feed should contain about 60–70 G protein, which will require a urine output of approximately 1,000–2,000 ml, implying a total fluid intake of 2,000–3,000 ml, to effect complete excretion.

According to Masterton *el al.* Ref. 4 (to whose paper reference should be made for further details) a 3,000 calorie diet for full nourishment could be made as follows:

Cows milk: 1,000 ml
50% Fat emulsion ('Prosparol'): 270 ml
Lactose: 250 G   } Total volume 2,970 ml
Milk protein ('Casilan'): 35 G
Water: 1,700 ml

The sodium content of this feed is 25 mEq and potassium 40 mEq. Extra vitamins together with sodium and potassium may be added as required, but excess sodium too may cause an osmotic diuresis. The feed must be made up only shortly before being given and with full hygenic precautions as it is an excellent culture medium for bacteria. It must never, therefore, be allowed to stand around at room temperature. It is generally given in divided doses four hourly.

Great attention must be paid to the accuracy of fluid balance charts on these patients and blood and urine sodium, potassium, urea and osmolality should be monitored regularly.

It bears emphasizing that the two most important complications of tube feeding are diarrhoea (which may be osmotic in nature due to too high an electrolyte or sugar content of the feed or to bacterial infection) and dehydration secondary to an osmotic diuresis caused by an excessive protein intake which may be contained in proprietary foods.

If 'Complan' is used for tube feeding to *maintain* nutrition, a daily intake of 220 G will supply 1,000 calories and a protein intake of 68 G. It should be made up in a concentration of NOT greater than 15 per cent and thus must be added to at least 1,300 ml of water. The daily fluid intake must in addition be made up by adding at least a further 1,000 ml of water.

Detection and Assay of Drugs

Many drugs are hydroxylated and conjugated in the liver, and excreted in the urine. As a result of these changes they are rendered less toxic and more soluble and hence are more rapidly excreted.

The detection by 'spot tests' of a drug either in its original form or as one of its metabolites constitutes an important biochemical investigation.

Spot test on casual urine specimens in out-patients serve as a useful check as to whether or not a patient is taking tablets which have been prescribed by the doctor.

If multiple drug therapy is being administered it is frequently possible to detect one drug in the presence of another by simple separation procedures but in more complex situations the differentiation may only be effected by paper or gas chromatography.

These tests are also of use if it is suspected that a patient may be secretly taking unprescribed drugs and also in the unconscious patient suspected of having been poisoned, though in this case in addition to catheterization for urine specimens both blood and gastric contents should be kept for analysis.

Drug tests of urine acquire particular importance in psychiatric patients both in mental hospitals and in out-patient departments.

Quantitative assay as opposed to qualitative identification of drugs in the urine is of rather limited value, and generally speaking, blood samples are necessary for quantitative work.

Many factors influence the blood level of a drug. These include the dose, route of administration (e.g. by mouth or intravenously), rate of absorption either as a characteristic of the drug or due to gastro-intestinal disease, whether or not the patient is fasting, the time after administration that the blood sample is taken, the presence of liver and renal disease, hereditarily determined variations in the ability to detoxicate the drug, and the effect of other concurrently administered drugs. It is sometimes not appreciated that the administration of other drugs *in the past* may, as a result of induction of the detoxication mechanisms in the liver continue to affect the rate of excretion of subsequently administered drugs for many months or even years. Thus the interpretation of blood levels of drugs is a most complex matter. Nevertheless increasing use of blood levels of drugs is made in the management of patients. It is in fact just because the matter is so complex that blood levels are required, for example in monitoring the treatment of epileptic patients on anticonvulsant therapy. It should be realized however that the matter is further complicated by the fact that some patients react differently both with regard to the therapeutic effect of drugs and to their toxic effects with *the same blood levels*. Thus a patient who manifests acute toxic symptoms on a normal dose of, say, phenytoin may either be intoxicated with high blood levels due to failure of the normal rate of detoxication or with low levels presumably on account of a particular sensitivity of the nervous system to the drug as the result of a 'constitutional pre-disposition'. Experience shows that this particular phenomenon is frequently highly specific towards one drug or one group of drugs.

Both spot tests in urine and blood assays require to be sent to laboratories specialising in the particular test in question.

Screening Tests for Inborn Errors of Metabolism

Hereditary metabolic disorders may present at any age and in a great variety of ways. Some may only be detected accidentally in later life on, say, routine urine examination, being entirely benign and symptomless, and others will only come to light after some 'stressing' incident such as, for example, the administration of a drug which is metabolized abnormally drawing attention to an enzyme system which is deficient. Many hereditary metabolic disorders however are obvious from birth. A number of clinical observations should raise the suspicion of an inborn error of metabolism. Examples are:

1. Any form of physical deformity including failure to thrive particularly if associated with mental deficiency;

2. Epilepsy of early onset;

3. Early development of cataracts;

4. Known metabolic disorders in, or unexplained early death of siblings;

5. Intolerance to certain types of food.

It is important, however, that diagnoses should be made as early as possible in life if effective treatment is to be given. Thus although routine urine testing of 'at risk' groups such as mentally defective children is vital, the aim should be to exclude metabolic disorders shortly after birth. This means that all infants should be tested with the full realization that only exceedingly rarely will an important case be picked up. *The continual finding of negative results therefore must not be allowed to predispose to careless testing.* Moreover, it is advisable to carry out tests on more than one occasion (vide infra).

The diagnosis of a metabolic disorder is not of course made on the basis of a positive 'spot' test, this being only an indication for further more detailed investigations. Most tests are performed on small amounts of urine and certain 'test papers' can be used on wet nappies. For some purposes a single drop of blood from a heel-prick is necessary, but the number of tests which can be applied is restricted, and thus they are by no means specific but 'merely screening' in nature, and if positive warrant further investigation of the patient. They are designed to give no false negative results though a few false positive results may occur from time to time but are clearly of no significance if adequately followed up and shown in fact not to be due to any serious disorder.

The World Health Organization has recently produced a pamphlet (Ref 5.) which may be consulted for further details.

A number of these tests can be carried out 'on the district' once the basic reagents have been made up, while all can be performed in clinical side-rooms of surgeries, post-natal clinics and hospital out-patient departments.

Practical details of tests for inborn errors of metabolism (from Buist. Ref. 6.)

TESTS ON URINE

[*Smell.* Characteristic odours have been reported in several metabolic diseases, and a summary of these is shown in Table 1. The odours are often most apparent in the urine, but the smell may be evanescent and difficult to describe and may be obscured by preservatives in the sample.

Table 1. *Diseases in which a specific smell has been described.*

Disease	Odour	Compound
Phenylketonria	Mouse-like	Phenylacetic acid
Maple syrup urine disease	Maple syrup. Sweetish	Branched chain. δ-Keto-acids
Methionine malabsorption	Sour berry smell. Reminiscent of a brewery	δ-Ketobutyric acid
Cystinuria	Sulphurous	Hydrogen sulphide
Homocystinuria	Sulphurous	Hydrogen sulphide
Isovaleric acidaemia	Sweaty feet. 'Cheesy"	Isovaleric acid
Green acyl dehydrogenase deficiency	Sweaty feet	Butyric acid. Hexanoic acid

Reducing substances. Reagent: Clinitest (Ames).
Method: Test according to manufacturer's instructions.

Reducing substances which may produce a positive Clinitest

Glucose: Diabetes mellitus, renal glycosuria, renal tubular dystrophies, Fanconi's syndrome, cystinosis, Lowe's syndrome, vitamin-D-resistant rickets (Dent type II).

Fructose: Fructosaemia (aldolase deficiency), essential fructosuria.

Galactose: Galactosaemia and variants, galactokinase deficiency.

Lactose: Lactase deficiency, congenital or acquired.

Xylulose: Pentosuria.

Homogentisic acid: Alkaptonuria.

Phenols: Phenylketonuria, tyrrosinosis, tyrosine transaminase deficiency.

Drugs: Ascorbic acid, chloral hydrate, sulphonamides, P.A.S., tetracycline, chloramphenicol.

Ferric chloride and Phenistix. Ferric chloride reagent—10 per cent aqueous ferric chloride. The reagent should be stored in a brown bottle in the refrigerator.

Method: Add two drops of reagent to 1 ml of urine. Mix and observe the colour immediately and 2–3 minutes later.

Phenistix: Test according to manufacturer's instructions.

[*Cyanide-nitroprusside (for sulphur-containing amino-acids)*. Reagents: (A) 5 per cent sodium cyanide. (B) 5 per cent aqueous sodium nitroferricyanide (sodium nitroprusside). (C) 2N sodium hydroxide. Reagents A and B should be stored in brown bottles in the refrigerator. Reagents A should be made freshly each month. Both solutions are dangerous and require caution in handling and storage.

Method: with pH paper alkalinize 2·5 ml of urine with reagent C to pH 6–8. Add 1 ml of reagent A to the urine. After mixing and standing for 20 minutes add one drop of reagent B.

Results: A pink-red or beet colour within 5 minutes indicates an abnormal urine. A false-negative result will occur if the urine is too acidic. The colour reaction is given by compounds which possess a free sulphydryl group or disulphide bond. Cystine and homocystine are therefore detected by the test, but cystathionine, methionine, and taurine do not react. The test is sensitive enough for even heterozygotes of cystinuria types 2 and 3 to give a positive result.]

Ninhydrin test (for excess amino-acids). Reagent: 1 G of ninhydrin dissolved in 500 ml of 95 per cent ethanol. The reagent should be kept in a dark bottle in the refrigerator.

Method: Add three drops of urine to 1 ml of reagent in a clean test-tube and mix. Examine for colour after 3-4 minutes.

Results: A blue or purple colour is taken to indicate the presence of excessive amino-aciduria, but a positive result may be caused by an

Table 2 *Diseases and compounds giving a reaction with ferric chloride and/or Phenistix*

	Ferric Chloride	Phenistix
Phenylketonuria	+ Blue-green	+
Tyrosine transaminase deficiency, tyrosinosis, tyrosuluria		
(p-hydroxyphenylpyruvic acid)	+Transient blue-green	+
*Histidinzemia	+/Œ Grey/green	+/Œ
Hyperglycinaemia	+/Œ Green	+
Maple syrup urine disease	+ Blue	+
(δ-ketoisovaleric acid)	+ Blue	+
(δ-ketoisocaproic acid)	Yellow	*
(δ-ketomethyl valeric acid)	Blue-green	*
Methionine malabsorption		
(δ-ketobutyric acid)	Purple fading to red/brown	+
Lactic acidosis	+/Œ Grey	+
Pyruvic acidaemia	Yellow	Yellow
Pyridoxine disorders, Kynureniniase deficiency		
(3-OH-anthranilic acid)	Immediate browm	Yellow
(xanthurenic acid)	Deep green × brown	—
Homogentisic acid	Transient blue-green	—
Acetoacetic acid	Brown/red	—
Conjugated bilirubin	Bluish green	*
Melanin	Grey precipitate × black	*
Salicylates	Purple	Purple
P.A.S.	Purple-brown	Purple
Isonicotinic acid hydrazide	Grey	*
Phenothiazines	Purple-brown	Purple
Phenols	Purple-brown	—
Vanillic acid	Red/brown-mauve	*

* Not tested.

artifact such as concentrated urine or a high ammonia content of the sample. Conversely, elevation of *single* amino-acids may not be detected by this method if the overall quantity of urinary amino-acids is not increased.

Ehrlich's Aldehyde (for porphobilinogen). See section on urine testing, Appendix D. p. 96.

Notes on Blood Groups and Blood Transfusion

Blood groups

There are numerous known blood group systems in the human. These include the ABO, Rhesus, Lewis, Kell, Duffy etc. systems. From the point of blood transfusion it is fortunate that only the first two are of major importance. It is therefore routine to establish only the ABO and Rhesus groups of a patient. With reference to the remaining groups if there is any incompatibility between the recipient and donor this will become apparent in the cross-matching process. Only in these circumstances would it be necessary to document the other groups.

The actual incidence of the different ABO groups varies at different geographical locations, and even within Great Britain there is a slight change from south to north. In general, however, the approximate incidence is shown in Table 1.

Certain combinations of antigens and antibody produces agglutination (see Table 3).

Table 3. *To show approximate incidence of blood groups in Great Britain.*

Group 0	50% of the population	Rh	85%
Group A	45% of the population	+ve	
Group B	12% of the population		
Group AB	3% of the population	Rh	15%
		−ve	

The blood group antigens are found in the red cells, and the antibodies in the serum (or plasma) (Table 2.)

Table 4. *To show nature of antigens and antibodies in different blood groups.*

ABO system	Antigens (in red cells)	Antibodies (in serum)
Group O	None	Anti-A and anti-B
Group A	A	Anti-B
Group B	B	Anti-A
Group AB	A and B	None

Table 5. *To show reaction of different ABO group antigens with anti-A and anti-B serum.*

	Anti-A	Anti-B
Group O	—	—
Goup A	+	—
Group B	—	+
Group AB	+	+

+ = agglutination   — = no agglutination.

This data is used in the laboratory tests for determining blood groups, and in the cross matching process.

When a patient has been grouped, bottles of that same group are selected for cross matching. There are, however, certain circumstances when other groups may be given, provided of course that the cross match does not detect any other incompatibility. It is even more vital to note that the circumstances denoted by NC are *NEVER* compatible (see Table 6).

Table 6. *To illustrate compatible and incompatible combinations of blood.*

Recipient Group	Donor O	A	B	AB
O	C	NC	NC	NC
A	C	C	NC	NC
B	C	NC	C	NC
AB	C	C	C	C

C = These are compatible provided that no other antigen-antibody reaction is detected by the cross-matching technique.
NC = NEVER COMPATIBLE.

Cross matching.

The details of the routine for this process varies slightly with different laboratories, but the basic principle is essentially the same, namely to detect any antibodies in the recipient's serum which may react with the cells from the proposed donor (taken from the pilot bottle, or in the case of plastic bags, directly from the tube connected to the bag).

In brief, the reaction is studied in tubes in the laboratory (i.e. *in vitro*) before being transfused to the patient (i.e. *in vivo*), by 3 different techniques.

1. In saline medium.
2. In albumin medium.
3. Indirect Coombs Test.

The latter is a very sensitive test which is able to detect antibodies which may not be found by the other two techniques.

Blood transfusion

Before setting up a blood transfusion it is essential to check carefully the number and expiry date of the bottle, the full name of the patient, hospital case number, blood group, age and ward. Haemolysed blood must not be used and blood must not be stored on the ward, but collected shortly before use and signed for in the laboratory. It is important to note that the ward staff are the last in line of an elaborate series of checks to ensure that the patient receives the correct bottle.

Blood transfusion is a potentially dangerous process and the patient's progress must be observed at intervals throughout, particularly for the first 15 minutes. It is the nurse's responsibility to report immediately any untoward reactions to the Sister in charge, in which case the transfusion should be stopped and the doctor in charge of the patient informed.

Transfusion hazards can be divided into:

1. Reaction of patient to the transfused blood.

2. Reaction of patient to overtransfusion (particularly important in elderly patients with cardiovascular diseases who are anaemic).

3. Toxic effect of potassium and citrate when large amounts of blood are given quickly.

4. Air embolism danger when transfusion is given under pressure.

5. Infection at site of needle or canula leading to thrombophlebitis.

6. Transmission of disease, e.g. homologous serum jaundice, malaria and some virus diseases.

7. Long term effects such as haemosiderosis when vast numbers of transfusions are given over a lengthy period (e.g. for patients with aplastic anaemia).

Transfusion reactions have a number of possible causes:

1. Infected blood (very serious).

2. Incompatible blood (very serious).

3. Allergy.

4. Pyrogens.

5. Haemolysed blood.

6. Over rapid transfusion.

Signs and symptoms to watch for:

1. Patient complains of feeling cold, shivery, pain in the back, difficulty in breathing.

2. Swelling of face.
3. Puffiness of eyelids.
4. Urticaria.
5. Temperature rise.
6. Pulse rise.
7. Rigor.
8. Distension of neck veins.

Investigation of transfusion reaction

1. Check blood group of pre-transfusion sample of patient's blood.

2. Check blood group of post-transfusion sample of patient's blood.

3. Check blood group of pilot bottle (if glass bottle is used).
4. Check blood group of blood from bottle or plastic pack.
5. Check cross match procedure.
6. Examine urine of patient for haemoglobinuria.
7. Blood urea.
8. Culture patient's blood.
9. Culture blood from bottle (or plastic bag.) at 37°C and 4°C.
10. Serum haptoglobins.
11. Direct Coombs test on post-transfusion blood sample
12. Schumm's test.

Further investigations with reference to other blood group systems (than ABO and Rhesus) may be necessary.

Blood containers

1. Plastic bags.
2. Glass bottles.

The advantage with the former is that a small sample of blood can be taken from the actual blood that will be transfused to the patient, without the risk of infection. This is done by filling one of the long tubes projecting from the bag with blood, placing a clip near the end of the tube, compressing it very firmly, and cutting off the distal end. This sample is then used to carry out the laboratory test. There is no way of taking a sample of blood from a glass bottle without the risk of contamination. For this reason there is always a small pilot bottle attached, which therefore has to be filled separately with the donor's blood.

Packed cells

Packed cells are sometimes requested for patients who are severely anaemic, and who therefore need a transfusion in order to restore the red cell volume, as opposed to whole blood volume which would need to be restored in a patient acutely shocked following a haematemesis. Packed cells would also be indicated in a patient in whom all unnecessary fluid was contraindicated, e.g. congestive cardiac failure, and in special rare cases where the plasma contains unwanted antibodies, and in which case only the cells would be transfused.

If packed cells are required, they may be supplied to the ward in plastic bags or in glass bottles. If in plastic bags, the life of the cells is the same as that of whole blood (i.e. three weeks is the commonly accepted interval from the date of donation), and there is no problem. If, however, a bottle is cross matched, the supernatant plasma has to be aspirated by the laboratory technician before being issued to the ward. There is one important proviso, namely that this must be done only just before the bottle leaves the laboratory. This transfusion should then commence immediately, as the bottle must be used within several hours, owing to the possibility of infection following aspiration procedure. If the bottle is not used within several hours it must be discarded.

Fresh blood transfusion

It is sometimes necessary to transfuse fresh blood (as opposed to stored blood) in the following conditions:

1. Where platelets are needed in a haemorrhagic disorder due to thrombocytopenia.

2. Haemophilia.

3. In the case of a rare blood group where stored blood of the required group may not be available. A donor might therefore have to be bled immediately prior to the transfusion.

Transfusion of platelets (Platelet rich plasma)
Indicated thrombocytopenic purpura. Must be used at once without storage.

Glossary of Medical and Technical Terms

A-β-lipoproteinaemia, a rare hereditary condition in which there is an absence of β-lipoprotein (a particular form of compound of lipid and protein) in the blood.

A-γ-globulinaemia, a rare condition of unknown cause in which there is an absence of free globulin in the blood.

acanthrocyte, an abnormal shape of red cell with thorny projections characteristically seen in A-β-lipoproteinaemia.

acidosis, a decrease in pH of the blood.

acromegaly, a chronic disease of adult life due to the elaboration of excessive growth hormone from an adenoma of the anterior pituitary and characterized by enlargement of the jaw, hands, feet and many organs.

Addisonian anaemia, see pernicious anaemia.

Addison's disease, a chronic disease of the adrenal gland sometimes due to tuberculosis resulting in deficient activity of the adrenal cortex.

adenoma, (e.g. chromophobe, eosinophil, basophil), a benign tumour of glandular tissue.

adrenal cortex, the outer part of the adrenal gland which produces hormones concerned with carbohydrate, water and electrolyte metabolism. It is essential to life.

adrenal medulla, the internal part of the adrenal gland which elaborates adrenaline. It is not essential to life.

adrenocorticotrophic hormone (A.C.T.H.), a hormone elaborated by the pituitary which stimulates the adrenal cortex.

adrenogenital syndrome, a congenital disorder in which there is an enzyme deficiency in the adrenal cortex which results in deficient cortisol production and certain masculinizing features in the female.

agglutination, the clumping together in characteristic fashion of red cells (for instance) when the appropriate antiserum (antibody) is added.

agranulocytosis, a state where there is a deficiency in the white cell series of the granulocyte cells (polymorpho-nuclear leucocytes).

aldosterone, a hormone of the adrenal cortex. It causes renal tubular retention of sodium and loss of potassium.

alimentary system, the digestive system.

alkali reserve, the base (i.e. compounds which combine with acid to form salts) which is held in combination in blood plasma. It is expressed in terms of carbon dioxide liberated by an acid.

alkalosis, an increase in pH of the blood.

alkaptonuria, a hereditary inborn error of metabolism in which there is an excretion in the urine of large amounts of homogentisic acid.

δ-amino-laevulinic acid, (A.L.A.) a metabolic precursor of porphobilinogen which appears in the urine of some patients with porphyria, it may be detected between attacks of acute intermittent porphyria.

amyloidosis, a degenerative condition which follows some chronic diseases often associated with the long standing presence of pus. It may follow tuberculosis.

There are extracellular deposits of an abnormal protein in the tissues particularly in the spleen, liver and kidney.

anaphylaxis, an acute reaction *in vivo* between an antigen and its antibody, leading to severe difficulty in breathing and collapse unless rapidly treated with adrenaline, hydrocortisone and antihistamines.

anisocytosis, variation of red cell size noted on a blood film, and found in iron deficiency and other anaemias.

ante-cutibal fossa, the depression in front of the elbow.

antibodies, these are the proteins in the serum which are either: 1. Naturally occurring (e.g. the anti-A in the plasma of group B patients), or 2. Immune, produced in the individual as a result of stimulation by blood group antigens not present in his or her own circulation but which have been introduced artificially (e.g. transfusion of blood of a different group).

antidiuretic hormone (A.D.H.) Vasopression. A hormone released by the posterior part of the pituitary gland which causes reabsorption of water by the renal tubules and reduces the volume of urine formed. Its absence results in diabetes insipidus.

antigens, Foriegn substances which when injected give rise to antibodies.

antihaemophilic globulin, a plasma protein; deficiency is responsible for the defect of coagulation in haemophilia.

antinuclear factor (A.N.F.), antibody found in the serum of patients with certain collagen diseases (e.g. Disseminated lupus erythematosus.)

basal metabolic rate (B.M.R.), the rate of the sum total of chemical changes which keep the body functioning and at a normal temperature while at complete rest.

base excess, the difference between the actual buffer base and the normal buffer base

Bence-Jones protein, an abnormal protein which appears in the urine in some cases of myelomatosis and rarely in chronic leukaemia. It dissolves on boiling the urine and re-precipitates on cooling.

biochemistry, the study of the chemical processes of living organisms and tissues.

biopsy, the taking of whole tissue samples at an operation or by needle, for histological or chemical examination.

buffer base, refers to non-volatile buffer ions and includes bicarbonate and proteinate in plasma and in addition heamoglobin in whole blood.

caeruloplasmin, an α_2 globulin which transports copper in the plasma. It exhibits oxidase activity (copper oxidase) and is deficient in Wilson's disease.

carcinoidosis, a tumour of the small gut which metastasises and produces characteristic symptoms on account of its secretion of 5-hydroxyptamine (5-H.T.) which is then excreted as 5-hydroxy-indole acetic acid (5-H.I.A.A.). Some lung tumours also secrete 5-H.T.)

carcinoma, a malignant tumour of epithelial tissue. The commonest form of cancer.

carcinomatosis, widespread secondary carcinoma.

catecholamines, the hormones of the adrenal medulla comprising chiefly adrenaline and nor-adrenaline. They are not essential to life.

christmas disease, a coagulation disorder of blood due to deficiency of christmas factor.

chromatography, a technique for the separation of chemical compounds usually of similar structure by virtue of their different mobilities on media impregnated with flowing solvents.

cirrhosis (of liver), progressive fibrosis as a result of disease with much tissue destruction and regeneration.

clearance tests, tests concerned with the measurement of the volume of blood theoretically completely cleared of a compound in unit time (usually 1 minute).

coeliac disease, a chronic disorder of childhood due to an intolerance to gluten in the diet resulting in a wasting disease with all the features of the malabsorption syndrome, and failure to thrive.

collagen, a protein occurring in the ground substance of connective tissue.

collagen diseases, disseminated lupus erythematosus, polyarteritis nodosa, scleroderma, dermatomyositis, temporal arteritis, rheumatoid arthritis. These condition are grouped together because of certain similar pathological changes in the tissue.

conjugation, the combination of one compound with another to form a product of biological importance. It often refers to the combination of drugs or their metabolites with glucuronic acid or sulphate to facilitate excretion by the kidneys.

Coombs test, direct—a test for antibodies attached to red cells. Indirect—a test for antibodies present in serum.

cortisol (hydrocortisone), the most important hormone secreted by the adrenal cortex. It is concerned with water, salt and carbohydrate metabolism and is essential to life.

Crohn's disease, a disease in which the small intestine undergoes a chronic inflammation and ulceration, leading eventually to obstruction. The cause is unknown.

cryoglobulin, an abnormal serum globulin which separates out of solution as a white precipitate on cooling.

Cushing's syndrome (disease), Cushing's syndrome is a clinical condition characterized by obesity, round face, pink striae of the skin, hypertension, osteoporosis, polycythaemia, amenorrhoea and hirsutism in females and decreased glucose tolerance. It is caused by a high circulating cortisol level. There are many causes one of which is a basophil tumour of the pituitary gland in which case the condition is called Cushing's disease.

cystic fibrosis of the pancreas (mucoviscidosis), a generalized inherited disorder of unknown cause in which there is dysfunction of the exocrine glands including the mucus secreting glands. It is primarily a disease of childhood but is now increasingly recognized in adults and is characterized by chronic pulmonary obstruction by viscid mucous, malabsorption, intestinal obstruction and high sweat sodium and chloride concentrations leading to sodium depletion and sometimes collapse in hot weather.

diabetes insipidus, (D.I.) a disorder caused by lack of vasopressin (antidiuretic hormone—A.D.H.) released from the posterior pituitary gland, it is characterized by the passing of large volumes of dilute urine and intense thirst.

diabetes mellitus, a disease in which there is an inability to metabolise glucose leading to high blood sugar levels, the excretion of large amounts of urine containing sugar and eventually to ketosis and coma. There are many causes but the definitive treatment lies in the administration of insulin.

diuretic, a drug which produces an increase of urine volume.

electrolyte, 1. A substance which dissolves in water with dissociation into ions, such a solution being capable of conducting an electric current. 2. The ionized salts of the blood including sodium, potassium, chloride and bicarbonate.

electrophoresis, an analytical technique in which charged colloidal particles (e.g. proteins) are separated by their relative motions towards electrodes placed in a buffered electrolyte medium.
Immunoelectrophoresis electrophoresis followed by precipitation with antibodies.

enzyme, protein compounds found throughout living tissues which in small amounts markedly accelerate biochemical reactions without themselves apparently being changed by these reactions. Co-enzyme, a non-protein compound necessary for enzyme activity.

erythropoiesis, the process of red cell production in the bone marrow.

(De-Toni) Fanconi syndrome, a rare congenital disorder resulting in multiple biochemical disorders many of which include abnormalities of the renal tubules such as impaired ability to reabsorb glucose, phosphate and amino-acids or to regulate the urine acidity.

ferritin, the soluble form of stored iron.

fibrinogen, a protein in plasma which is converted to fibrin during the process of blood coagulation.

fibrosis, a reaction of tissue particularly in response to infection involving excess production of fibroblasts and collagen.

formiminoglutamic acid F.I.G.L.U., a metabolite of histidine which accumulated in abnormal amounts in folic acid deficiency.

Friedreich's ataxia, a familial disease beginning in early life characterized by unsteadiness of gait and abnormal reflexes due to disease of the posterior and lateral columns of the spinal cord.

function tests, biochemical function tests are investigations designed to estimate the efficiency and degree of reserve function in a particular system or organ. Examples include renal, liver, endocrine, gastric and respiratory function tests.

galactosaemia, an inborn error of metabolism due to an enzyme deficiency in red cells which results in a rise of blood galactose and a low blood sugar after milk feeds, jaundice a failure to thrive and mental deficiency in later life if untreated.

glomerulus (renal), a structure lying within the outer part of the kidney (cortex) containing a tuft of small blood vessels which filters fluid from the blood which after concentration in the kidney tubules gives rise to urine.

glucagon, a hormone derived from the pancreas which results in the breakdown of liver glycogen and a rise of blood sugar.

glycogen, animal starch which is stored in the tissues particularly the liver, spleen and muscle and which serves as a reserve store of carbohydrate.

glycogen storage disease, rare hereditary disorders in which there is an enzyme deficiency resulting in metabolic abnormalities characterized by abnormal accumulation of glycogen in the tissues. They are often subdivided into those in which the glycogen is deposited throughout many tissues in the body (general glycogenosis) and those in which it is mainly deposited in muscle (muscle glycogenosis).

gonadotrophins (pituitary), hormones derived from the anterior part of the pituitary gland which stimulate the testis and ovary. During pregnancy chorionic gonadotrophin is derived from the placenta.

growth hormone (somatotrophin), a hormone elaborated by the anterior part of the pituitary gland which promotes normal growth. Excess production result in gigantism before puberty and acromegaly after puberty.

haematology, the study of blood disorders.

haemochromatosis, a condition mainly confined to males in which there is excessive absorption of iron and excessive deposition in the tissues.

haemoglobinopathies, diseases due to chemically abnormal haemoglobins.

haemoglobinuria, the presence of haemoglobin in the urine.

haemophilia, a disease in which there is defective blood coagulation due to deficiency of a specific circulating globulin (antihaemophilic globulin).

haemolytic anaemias, result from an increased rate of red cell destruction.

haemosiderin, the insoluble form of storage iron.

haemosiderosis, a condition in which there is deposition of haemosiderin compound in tissues particularly liver and spleen due to increased rate of destruction of red cells.

haptoglobins, proteins in the plasma which combine with and remove small amounts of free haemoglobin.

Henoch Schönlein purpura, an allergic purpura commonly associated with acute infections of the throat.

Hepatitis, inflammation of the liver.

heterozygote, one inheriting different characteristics from each parent.

hirsutism, a term referring to an excessive growth and abnormal distribution of hair particularly in the female.

histamine, an amine found widely distributed in the tissues. When injected it produces many of the clinical features of allergy.

homogentisic acid, an acid not normally detectable in the urine which is present in high concentration in patients with almaptonuria. It gives a positive reaction for reducing substances in the urine and at the same time turns the urine black. The specific test for glucose is of course negative.

homozygote, one inheriting the same characteristics from each parent.

hormone, a physiologically active compound secreted by the endocrine glands.

11-hydroxycorticosteroids, a group of hormones derived from the adrenal cortex which are concerned with sodium, water and carbohydrate metabolism. They include cortisol and some similar compounds but exclude a number of its precursors.

17-hydroxycorticosteroids, a group of hormones derived from the adrenal cortex which are concerned with sodium, water and carbohydrate, metabolism. They include cortisol and many of its precursors.

5-hydroxyindole acetic acid (5HIAA), a metabolite of 5-hydroxytryptamine which is excreted in the urine in excessive amounts in patients with carcinoidosis.

hydroxylation, a chemical transformation involving the substitution of an (-OH-) group into a molecule.

5-hydroxytryptamine, a biologically active amine present in high concentration in the small intestinal mucosa. It is secreted in large amounts by carcinoid tumours and gives rise to excretion of increased concentrations 5-hydroxyindole acetic acid in the urine.

hyperglycaemia, a concentration of glucose in the blood above the upper limit of normal.

hypernatraemia, a concentration of sodium in the blood above the upper limit of normal.

hyperplasia, a condition in which there is an increase in the number of cells in an organ or tissue.

hypertension, persistently abnormally high arterial blood pressure and the associated changes in the heart and blood vessels.

hyperthyroidism, over activity of the thyroid gland.

hypertonic, in medical terminology refers to a solution having an osmotic pressure greater than that of normal plasma.

hypogammaglobulinaemia, a state which there is a decrease in the free circulating globulin in the blood. It is secondary to a number of conditions some of which are associated with a decrease in all protein fractions.

hypoglycaemia, blood sugar below the lower limit of normal.

hypophosphatasia, a deficiency of alkaline phosphatase.

hypokalaemia, blood potassium below the lower limit of normal.

idiopathic, relating to a condition of unknown cause.

immunoglobulins, proteins which have antibody activity.

infarction, the production of an area of dead tissue due to obstruction of blood supply in an end artery.

insulinoma, a tumour of the pancreas which secretes insulin. It may be benign or malignant.

intrinsic factor, a protein in the gastric juice the presence of which is necessary for combination with vitamin B_{12} in the process of its absorption. It is deficient in pernicious anaemia and after partial gastrectomy.

iso-enzymes, a family of enzymes with similar properties which are usually separable by electrophoresis.

isotonic, refers to solutions which exert equal osmotic pressures.

isotopes, elements which have the same atomic number but different atomic weights. Isotopes of an element share the same chemical properties; thus those isotopes which are radioactive can be used as 'labels' for following chemical and biochemical reactions which normally involve the stable isotopes.

ketosis, the presence of excessive ketones in the body fluids and tissues found in states of severe starvation particularly if associated with prolonged vomiting, and in diabetic coma.

kwashiorkor, a condition of chronic malignant malnurition in children seen mostly in tropical Africa and the West Indies. ↘ *England, Uk*

lactic acidosis, a disorder in which there is an excessive accumulation of lactic acid in the blood.

latex test, polystyrene latex or polyvinyl toluene latex particles are coated with antigen. When mixed with serum containing the antibody clumping of the particles occurs. Many antibodies can be detected by this method.

lupus erythematosus cells—L.E. cells, characteristic cells found *in vitro* testing of blood from a patient with lupus erythematusus. They are not found circulating in the blood (*in vivo*.)

Lesh–Nyhan syndrome, an exceedingly rare congenital disorder characterized clinically by mental deficiency and abnormal movements with a tendency to self-destructive mutilation particularly of the mouth, and biochemically by extremely high serum uric acid and a high renal excretion of uric acid.

leukaemias, an abnormal proliferation of the leucocytes characterized by production of excess numbers of the more primitive precursor cells. There are many different types of leukaemia—the actual predominant cells varying with the type.

lipids, fatty compounds which occur in living tissues.

lymphoma, tumours arising from the cells of lymphoid tissue.

macrocytic anaemia, anaemia in which large red cells (macrocytes) are present in the peripheral blood film. It is characteristic of a number of conditions but particularly vitamin B_{12} and folate deficiency.

macroglobulinaemia, the presence in blood of an abnormal globulin having a high molecular weight. It is formed in some diseases of the bone marrow and lymphatic systems.

malabsorption syndrome, a group of conditions characterized by impairment of normal intestinal absorption of many dietary constituents but especially of fats and fat soluble vitamins and generally associated with multiple features of malnutrition including failure to develop normally when present in childhood.

mean (arithmetic), the average of a series of numbers.

mean corpuscular haemoglobin (M.C.H.), average mass of haemoglobin in each red cell ($\mu\mu$g). Calculated as follows:
$$10 \times \text{haemoglobin (G/100 ml)} \div \text{red cell count (millions per cmm)}$$

mean corpuscular haemoglobin concentration (M.C.H.C.), average concentration of haemoglobin in red cells (%). Calculated as follows:
$$100 \times \text{haemoglobin in G/100 ml} \div \text{packed cell volume (\%)}$$

mean corpuscular volume (M.C.U.), mean volume of red cells expressed in cubic microns ($c\mu$). Calculated as follows:
$$10 \times \text{P.C.V. (\%)} \div \text{red cell count (millions per cmm)}$$

measurement—units

Volume   1 litre (L)   = 1,000 millilitres (1,000 ml)

             1 millilitre (ml)   = 1,000 microlitres (1,000 μl)

Weight   1 kilogram (kg)   = 1,000 grams (1,000 g)

             1 gram (g)   = 1,000 milligrams (1,000 mg)

             1 milligram (mg) = 1,000 micrograms (1,000 μg)

             1 milliequivalent $\equiv$ equivalent weight in milligrams.

In clinical biochemistry most constituents are expressed in mg/100 ml or mEq/L.

$$mEq/L = \frac{mg/100\ ml \times 10 \times valency}{atomic\ weight}$$

To convert concentrations of the following in mg/100 ml to mEq/l divide by the appropriate factor.

         Bicarbonate—Expressed as vols/100 ml $\div$ 2·24

         Calcium $\div$ 2

         Chloride—Expressed as sodium chloride $\div$ 5·85

         Chloride—Expressed as chloride $\div$ 3·55

         Magnesium $\div$ 1·2

         Potassium $\div$ 3·9

         Sodium $\div$ 2·3

         Phosphate—Expressed as mgP/100 ml $\div$ 1·72.

megaloblastic, the type of erythropoiesis characterised by changes in the nuclei and cytoplasm of the red cell precursors in the bone marrow, and typical of either vitamin B_{12} or folate deficiency.

metabolism, the biochemical processes of life.

metachromatic material, Intracellular granules in urine deposit which stain characteristically for sulphatide.

metopirone, a drug which inhibits the production of cortisol by the adrenal cortex thus stimulating the pituitary to elaborate A.C.T.H., the effect of which is to increase *cortisol precursors* compounds from the adrenal cortex in the urine. Used as a test of pituitary function.

milk alkali syndrome, a syndrome caused by the excessive intake of milk and soluble alkali. Differentiation from hyperparathyroidism may be difficult.

myeloid metaplasia, the formation of marrow tissue in the spleen and liver, as a compensatory process in certain conditions when the bone marrow is unable to function properly.

myelomatosis, a malignant tumour which disseminates in the bone marrow and which is associated with destruction of bone, anaemia, abnormal plasma proteins and Bence-Jones protein in the urine.

myoglobin, muscle protein.

myoglobinuria, the presence of myoglobin in urine, following muscle destruction as in crush injuries.

McArdle's disease, a rare hereditary metabolic disorder caused by a deficiency of an enzyme (phosphorylase) in muscle and characterized by weakness and pain in limb muscles associated with abnormal accumulation of muscle glycogen and sometimes with myoglobinuria.

necrosis, death of tissue.

nephritis (type 1) (acute—chronic), an acute inflamatory disorder of unknown cause (probably allergic) of the glomeruli followed by widespread degenerative changes in the kidney. It often follows streptococcal infections of the throat and is associated with high blood pressure, oedema, impaired kidney function together with blood in the urine, most patients recover completely.

nephrotic syndrome (nephrosis) (e.g. type II nephritis), a syndrome caused by disease of the renal tubules and characterized by marked oedema, large quantities of protein in the urine, changes in the plasma proteins and a rise in plasma cholesterol. There are many causes including primary renal disease, collagen diseases and drug toxicity.

neuroblastoma, a malignant tumour of the adrenal medulla and autonomic nervous system which is usually seen in early childhood.

normal (solutions), in the physiological context (not chemical); a normal solution is one having the same osmotic pressure as plasma.

normoblastic, refers to normal blood formation in the bone marrow.

normochromic, normal degree of staining of the red cells on a blood film.

osmolality, a term referring to the measurement of osmotic pressure which is that pressure exerted by substances in solution particularly if highly dissociated (e.g. electrolytes) and which under certain circumstances may be used as a measure of the total amount of dissolved materials.

osmotic pressure, the pressure exerted by substances in solution through a semi-permeable membrane (i.e. a membrane which allows the passage through it of a solvent but not of the substances in solution).

osteomalacia, a generalized disorder of bone calcification which results in deformities due to softening of bones (adult rickets). There are many causes which in common give rise to deficient concentrations of calcium and phosphate in bone. These include dietary deficiency of calcium and vitamin D, renal tubular losses of phosphate and malabsorption syndromes.

osteoporosis, rarefaction of bone due to a deficiency of bone protein structure. Changes in bone calcium are secondary. It may be generalized or localized.

17-oxogenic steroids (17-ketogenic steroids), a group of hormones derived from the adrenal cortex which are concerned with sodium, water and carbohydrate metabolism. They include cortisol and many of its precursors.

17-oxosteroids (17-ketosteroids), a group of hormones derived from the adrenal cortex and the testis.

packed cell volume (P.C.V.) (haematocrit), the volume of packed red cells (ml per 100 ml) expressed as a percentage of the volume of blood in which they are contained.

Paget's disease of bone, a chronic disease of bone in elderly subjects in which there is a disorganization of bone structure characterized by softening of bone followed by thickening of bone cortex the cause is unknown.

pentagastrin, A synthetic compound which stimulates gastric secretion. Its action is similar to that of the natural hormone, gastrin.

pernicious anaemia (addisonian anaemia), a condition in which there is impairment of vitamin B_{12} absorption due to a lack of intrinsic factor in the gastric juice.

pH, the negative logarithm of the hydrogen ion concentration. It is an index of acidity-alkalinity, solutions having a pH below 7·0 being acidic and those above 7·0 alkaline.

phaeochromocytoma, a primary tumour of the adrenal medulla which forms adrenaline and allied compounds and which characteristically gives rise to paroxysmal hypertension.

phosphorylase, an enzyme present in tissues which accelerates the breakdown of glycogen.

plasma, the fluid portion of the blood in which the cells are suspended. It is obtained when whole blood is treated with an anti-coagulant to prevent clotting and the cells removed by centrifugation. It contains fibrinogen.

poikilocytosis, variation in shape of red cells noted on a blood film, and found e.g. in pernicious anaemia.

polycythaemia, an increase in the number of red cells per unit volume of blood.

polycythaemia rubra vera, a blood disease in which there is an excess of red cells in the circulation.

polyuria, abnormally large excretion of urine.

porphobilinogen, a non-fluorescent compound which is a metabolite of blood pigments. Its excretion in urine is markedly increased during attcks of acute intermittent porphyria.

porphyria, a group of disorders which may present clinically in a variety of ways, characterized by the presence of very high concentrations of porphyrins in the tissues and body fluids. Acute attacks may be precipitated by many factors including drugs, particularly barbiturates and sulphonamides, during which the urine contains fluorescent compounds.

porphyrins (uroporphyrins, coproporphyrins), fluorescent compounds with no known metabolic function in man derived from certain blood pigments. They are excreted in increased amounts in a number of conditions but in especially high concentrations in porphyria.

pregnanetriol, a hormone derived from the adrenal cortex which is normally present in small amounts in urine but which is excreted in very large amounts in the adrenogenital syndrome.

proteinuria, the presence of protein in the urine. Orthostatic proteinuria is a harmless condition seen in fit young adults in which protein appears in the urine after prolonged standing and disappears when urine collection is made after lying recumbent.

pseudocholinesterase, an enzyme present in tissues and plasma which splits compounds combined with choline, (c.f. true cholinesterase which inactivates acetyl choline at the neuromuscular junction and which is not present in plasma).

pseudohypoparathyroidism, a hereditary condition in which the biochemical abnormalities of hypoparathyroidism exist due to an insensitivity to parathyroid hormone. Bone deformities are also usually present.

psychogenic water drinking, a rare syndrome seen in patients with severe psychiatric disorders in which there is a desire to drink excessive quantities of water resulting in the passage of a large volume of urine.

purpura (petechiae), small pin point haemorhages in the skin.

pyelonephritis (chronic), a chronic slowly progressive disorder of uncertain cause presenting usually in late middle life with increasing renal impairment and often associated chronic infection of the urine.

pyloric stenosis, a thickening of the distal end of the stomach resulting in impaired passage of stomach contents into the duodenum.

pyrogen, a substance formed by micro-organisms which causes a rise of temperature when injected.

radioimmunoassay, a technique for the measurement of extremely small quantities of material (usually peptide hormones) which depends upon the measurement of the degree of binding of a radioactive labelled peptide with its antiserum under specific conditions.

Refum's disease, a familiar disorder characterised by an abnormal pigmentation of the retina, nerve deafness, chronic polyneuritis and skin lesions in which an increased level of phytanic acid has been detected in the serum and tissues.

renal failure, failure of kidney function.

reticulocyte, a red cell present in the circulation characterized by staining reactions which indicate it has recently been released from the bone marrow.

rickets, a disease of childhood in which there is softening and deformity of bones due to deficiency of vitamin D. There are however many causes of rickets other than dietary deficiency including malabsorption syndromes, renal failure, renal tubular disorders, cystinosis and resistance to the action of vitamin D.

rigor, a severe response to infections (e.g. malaria and renal disease) typified by uncontrollable shivering, feeling cold, and a sharp rise of temperature.

Rose-Waaler test, a serum test which becomes positive in patients with rheumatoid arthritis.

sarcoidosis, a generalized disease of unknown cause which manifests itself in many organs and particularly the skin, lungs, liver, spleen and nervous system. Histologically it produces characteristic lesions known as granulomas.

sarcoma, a malignant tumour of connective tissue.

Schilling test, a test of vitamin B_{12} absorption using oral administration of the radioactive vitamin as marker.

sedimentation rate, the rate at which suspended red cells settle when blood is allowed to stand under standard conditions. It is measured in mm per hour.

serum, the fluid portion of the blood which remains after whole blood is allowed to clot and the cells removed by centrifugation. It is very similar to plasma in many aspects but does not contain fibrinogen.

Sia tests, 1 drop of serum added to 100 ml deionized water causes a white precipitate in cases of macroglobulinaemia. The test is not specific.

spectroscopy, white light passed through a prism forms a spectrum of colours (from red at one end to blue at the other). If a sample (e.g. a dilute haemoglobin solution) is interposed it will absorb certain wavelengths and dark lines appear at characteristic positions in the spectrum. These lines allow certain pigments to be identified by their position.

standard bicarbonate, the concentration of bicarbonate in plasma from whole blood which has been equilibrated at 38°C at a PCo_2 of 40 mm Hg and with oxygen to give full saturation of the haemoglobin.

standard deviation, the standard deviation is a measure of the spread of numerical values about a mean value. It is defined as the square root of the mean of the squared deviations from the arithmetic mean of the distribution.

steatorrhoea, a condition in which there is an excess of fat in the stools.

sulphatides, a group of sulphur containing lipids occurring in particularly high concentration in myelin and therefore in white matter of the brain and spinal cord.

target cells, red cells found for example in certain haemoglobinopathies. The typical cell has a rim of normally staining haemoglobin within which is an area of diminished or no staining, and a central area of staining.

tetany, a state of increased neuromuscular excitability due to a decrease in the serum calcium or to alkalosis. Rarely it may be associated with a low serum magnesium.

thiamine pyrophospate, a co-enzyme essential for tissue intermediary metabolism of carbohydrates. It is derived from vitamin B_1.

thrombocythaemia, production of excess number of platelets.

thrombophlebitis, inflammation of the veins, often caused by bacterial organisms or sterile chemical irritation.

thyrotrophin (T.S.H. thyroid stim. hormone), a hormone elaborated by the anterior pituitary gland which stimulates the thyroid gland.

thyroxine, a hormone elaborated by the thyroid gland in response to TSH.

tolerance tests, tests in which an organ is 'stressed' biochemically in order to assess its degree of reserve function.

transketolase, an enzyme present in human red and white blood cells but not in the plasma. Its activity depends on the presence of thiamine pyrophosphate for which it is a sensitive test. `

tri-iodothyronine, a hormone elaborated by the thyroid gland. Its action is potent and rapid but it is only present in low concentrations in the bloodstream. It may be administered to patients therapeutically or used as an agent for suppressing the thyroid in diagnostic tests.

trimesters of pregnancy, the usual nine month period of pregnancy divided into 3 three month periods (trimesters).

tryptophan, an amino acid which is essential for growth and maintenance of health.

tubules (renal), part of the kidney which selectively absorbs certain constituents from the glomerular filtrate in the production of urine.

ulcerative colitis, a severe ulcerative condition of the colon of unknown cause characterized by fever, anaemia, and the passage in the stools of blood, mucus and pus.

ultracentrifugation, very high speed centrifugation used for separation of high molecular weight constituents. In diagnostic biochemical studies it is frequently used for separation of protein or lipid.

uraemia, the clinical and biochemical state which arises as a result of renal failure.

urticaria, skin manifestations of allergy. These are typically small raised itchy blebs over a large area of the body.

Van den Bergh reaction, a test for bilirubin in the serum.
　　　　　　　　direct positive＝Conjugated bilirubin
　　　　　　　　indirect positive＝Unconjugated bilirubin.

vanillymandelic acid (V.M.A.), (H.M.M.A.), one of the major metabolic products of catecholamines which is excreted in increased amounts in patients with phaeochromocytoma.

vasopression (antidiuretic hormone) (A.D.H.), a hormone derived from the posterior pituitary which promotes the re-absorption of water by the kidney tubules, absence of which gives rise to pituitary diabetes insipidus.

vitro (in), with reference to samples and specimens examined in the laboratory.

vivo (in), with reference to examinations involving the whole organism.

Wernicke's encephalopathy, a disorder due to deficiency of vitamin B_1 often seen in alcoholic patients characterized by disturbances of eye movement, unsteadiness of gait, confusion and peripheral neuritis.

Wilson's disease, a hereditary disorder in young people characterized by cirrhosis of the liver, degeneration of the basal ganglia of the brain and pigmented rings in the periphery of the iris of the eye (Kayser-Fleischer rings). There is a deficiency of caeruloplasmin in the plasma, a low serum copper and a high urine excretion of copper.

xanthinuria, a rare hereditary disease in which an enzyme deficiency (xanthine oxidase) is responsible for an abnormality in uric acid metabolism.

xanthine oxidase, an enzyme which converts hypoxanthine to xanthine and xanthine to uric acid. It is deficient in xanthinuria.

xanthochromia, yellowish discolouration generally used in reference to the cerebrospinal fluid which has been in contact with blood following subarachnoid haemorrhage.

xanthomatosis, firm tumours of lipid material which appear in the skin and tendon sheaths, in a number of conditions in which there is a high lipid content in the blood.

xylose, a sugar often used as a test for intestinal absorption of carbohydrate.

Zollinger-Ellison syndrome, a rare condition in which there is a very marked over secretion of hydrochloric acid by the stomach. This is associated with severe and multiple peptic ulcers and is due to a tumour of the pancreas which releases a factor responsible for stimulating the gastric secretion.

Selected References for
Further Reading

1. *Using the laboratory. A handbook for medical practitioners prepared on the advice of the standing Medical Advisory Committee and the Central Pathology Committee.* May 1970. (Department of Health and Social Security, Ref. G/H118/D)
2. DOREEN JACKSON, DAVID B. GRANT, BARBARA E. CLAYTON. 'A simple oral test of growth-hormone secretion in children', *Lancet* 1968, **2**, 373.
3. *Notes on clinical side-room methods, prepared by the subcommittee in medicine of the Medical Education Committee Edinburgh*, second edition, 1966 (E. and S. Livingstone Ltd.).
4. J. P. MASTERTON, H. A. F. DUDLEY, SHEILA MACRAE. 'Design of tube feeds for surgical patients', *British Medical Journal*, 1963, **2**, 909.
5. *Screening for inborn errors of metabolism.* Report of a W.H.O. scientific group. World Health Organisation Technical Report, September 1968 No. 401.
6. N. R. M. BUIST. 'Set of simple side-room urine tests for detections of inborn errors of metabolism', *British Medical Journal*, 1968, **2**, 745.

Index

NOTES

NOTES

NOTES

NOTES